But You Look So Good . . .
Stories by Carcinoid Cancer Survivors

Universe books may be ordered through booksellers or by contacting:

Universe LLC
63 Liberty Drive
Bloomington, IN 47403
www.iuniverse.com
1-800-Authors (1-800-288-4677)

ISBN: 978-1-4759-8131-5 (sc)
ISBN: 978-1-4759-8134-6 (ebk)

Printed in the United States of America
First Edition

iUniverse rev. date: 08/17/2013

BUT YOU LOOK SO GOOD

STORIES BY CARCINOID CANCER SURVIVORS

MARIA J. GONZAL

iUniverse LLC
Bloomington

I refuse to live a shadow of a life that could have been.

—Michael Huskey, Life Coach
www.theliferocket.com

The Aphorism

"Zebra" is a medical slang term for a surprising diagnosis.

The term derives from the aphorism *"When you hear hoof beats, don't look for zebras",* coined in the late 1940s by Dr. Theodore Woodward, a former professor at the University of Maryland School of Medicine in Baltimore, Maryland.[†]

Since horses are the most commonly encountered animal with hooves, and zebras are rare, one could confidently guess that the animal's hoofbeats are probably those of a horse. This generally applies to diagnosing diseases as well.

The Warning

In diagnosing the cause of illness in individual cases, calculations of probability have no meaning. The pertinent question is whether the disease is present or not. Whether it is rare or common does not change the odds in a single patient.

If the diagnosis can be made on the basis of specific criteria, then these criteria are either fulfilled or not.[††]

[†]Sotos, John G. (2006) [1991]. Zebra Cards: An Aid to Obscure Diagnoses. Mt. Vernon, VA: Mt. Vernon Book Systems. ISBN 978-0-9818193-0-3.

[††]Harvey, A. M., et al (1979). Differential Diagnosis (3rd ed.). Philadelphia: W.B. Saunders

Contents

Acknowledgments

In honor of all those living with neuroendocrine cancer and in memory of all who have gone before, especially the loss of our beloved Steve Jobs and John Thomas, owner of Wendy's restaurant chain. May we serve as their voice for a disease that is powerful, cunning, and sly.

In appreciation of the dedicated physicians who care for us, as well as all who are researching pathways to combat neuroendocrine cancer. A special thank you to Drs. M. Adler, P. Eastman, E Liu, T. O'Dorisio, L.Pia, R. Pommier, E. Woltering, and H. Jensen-Male, R.N.

This book is dedicated to all who are living with cancer, and the caregivers who generously contributed their personal stories.

Thank you A. Martin, D.Anderson, and B. Manewal for your generous time in editing, support, and guidance. Thank you Lucy Wiley for the idea for this book!

A heartfelt thank you to all who contributed in making this book come to fruition. You know who you are, and I share my heart and thoughts as friends!

Preface

The stories you are about to read are personal journeys that allow the reader to share the path from early onset of symptoms to the eventual diagnosis of carcinoid, under the umbrella of neuroendocrine cancer. Each journey is unique as this cancer is quite uncommon, YET MOST WILL share the common bonds of misdiagnosis, confusion, and uncertainty. Many, if not most, health care providers will never see a case in a lifetime of clinical practice.

I had practiced internal medicine and endocrinology for thirty years in a hospital based clinic and was familiar with the clinical features of carcinoid. However, despite treating thousands of patients during this time, I was unable to confirm a suspected case. That is, until Maria Gonzalez, my trusted colleague and co-worker in the diabetes and endocrine clinics described some personal symptoms that were nonspecific, such as weight loss, abdominal discomfort, and flushing.

An intense episode of abdominal and flank pain led to a CT scan showing low density lesions in the liver and a liver biopsy was consistent with a neuroendocrine tumor. The laboratory tests supported the diagnosis of carcinoid, and she, AS A BREAST CANCER SURVIVOR, was now faced with her second major health challenge. When you read her and other's stories in this book, you can imagine the many road blocks and speed bumps faced by those afflicted WITH this cancer. The treatment options are improving but optimal care often requires visits to academic medical centers in distant cities and countries. Local and internet-based support groups have evolved and have become invaluable in educating patients and families on the latest approaches to monitoring and treatment.

It is my hope that those who have openly shared their personal journeys in this book will have expanded our understanding of carcinoid for patients, care partners, and clinicians. This may lead to earlier diagnosis and more effective management. I wholeheartedly support the efforts of THESE CONTRIBUTORS.

—Martin E. Adler, M.D, Endocrinology and Internal Medicine

When my colleague Maria Gonzalez and I first met J., she had come to us as a referral from her primary care provider in a nearby city as no one could come up with a diagnosis of her complex assortment of symptoms which were very debilitating to her.

J. presented with profuse, malodorous steatorrhea (fatty stools, due malabsorption of fats), bloating, gas, significant weight loss and multiple arthralgias (joint pains), muscle pain and multiple neuropathies. She was having, on average, 20 or more stools per day and was living on Imodium until we started her on Lomotil˙. We eventually switched her to tincture of opium, the only medication which was able to control her diarrhea. We combined the tincture with octreotide rescue injections. With the use of these agents, she was able to reduce her stooling to 2-3 per day. We eventually started her on Sandostatin LAR® on a monthly basis.

I have had very thorough training in medical school, internship, and residency to become a hematologist and a medical oncologist. I had cared for many people in Vietnam during the height of the war and in Ethiopia with the Peace Corp. I had practiced for 40 years at our local county hospital in Northern California but had never seen a case of carcinoid until I met J.

We started her on Sandostatin˙, after consulting with our group's endocrinologist. He suggested the work-up for her symptoms and indeed, her 5-HIAA (a crucial test for the diagnosis of NETs) was very abnormal. We also checked a Chromogranin A (CgA). This test is one of the most important, both for diagnosis and monitoring of NE cancers. level, which was also abnormal. She was started on three-times-daily subcutaneous injections of octreotide which she self-administered and eventually the long acting analog, Sandostatin LAR˙. She continued the injections on a monthly basis with dose adjustment according to her symptoms.

The response to octreotide was immediate, and for once in a very long while, this vital woman was able to live her life outside of her bathroom and have some quality of life. Her family had rejected her, believing she was "putting on a show". She painfully described the lack of intimacy due to her symptoms, causing her boyfriend to abandon her.

After a colonoscopy revealed no pathology, we referred her to one of our surgeons who performed an exploratory laparotomy, leading to a bowel resection.

The patient was able to return home and did well for a few years on her monthly injections until she presented again with weight loss, anorexia, and profound fatigue. We admitted J. to our Long Term Care Unit as she had nowhere to go; no family members were willing to take her into their homes, and we decided that the most logical place for her was in a place where she would receive hospice care, surrounded by medical staff who would tend to her physical and spiritual needs. She died peacefully from complications of a line sepsis and bowel ischemia (lack of blood) to her intestine.

Caring for people with all cancers is a daunting task for any oncologist, but some are more complex than others. Carcinoid is in that category. J's initial presentation was mysterious: a challenge which drove me to research possible causes. I had the clinical intuition to consider carcinoid in my differential diagnosis, but nonetheless, I had to teach myself and my colleagues about this cancer.

All of us in medicine should be open-minded enough to always look beyond the obvious when we are taking a patient history. We do not want to miss a cancer that so profoundly affects people's lives. We need to teach our young providers that this is one cancer that must not be overlooked. In medical school we are taught to start with the most likely diagnosis: to look for horses, not zebras when we hear hoof beats, but with this cancer, one looks for and finds a zebra. In the case of NE cancers, no stone should be left unturned in pursuing the diagnosis.

Carcinoid disease can mimic so many other disease entities such as irritable bowel syndrome, ulcerative colitis, Crohn's disease, anxiety, depression, malingering and even Munchausen's. We must not let these other diseases throw us off track, thereby, causing a grave disservice to our patients.

In 2006, the Institute of Medicine published a landmark report titled "From Cancer Patient to Cancer Survivor: Lost in Transition."

I note this, since many patients with carcinoid live long lives with adequate symptom management by an expert in the field or the interested and informed oncologist. There are 10 million plus long-term cancer survivors in this country. The report underscores the staggering observation that these cancer survivors remain largely underserved, with many lost to medical follow-up entirely. Thanks to Lance Armstrong, Olivia Newton John, Sheryl Crow and Melissa Etheridge, public awareness has been boosted.

One of the most vexing and least discussed challenges for clinicians addresses reaching and educating long-term cancer survivors. Were it not for online groups that deal exclusively with supporting carcinoid cancer survivors, this group of patients would be severely neglected.

The patient with carcinoid lives with the ever-present possibility of recurrence, life-threatening crises when facing minor to major procedures, side effects of drugs, other malignancies, and being labeled as drug—seeking for the chronic pain syndrome associated with the disease.

Patients themselves are not aware of the possibility of a second malignancy, side effects of medications, or treatment options. If it were not for grass roots support groups and conferences where patients and providers come together to discuss this cancer, we would still be in the dark ages with this malignancy. It must be appreciated as a malignancy and not some disease that is either deemed indolent enough not to worry about, or that will spontaneously go into remission, although many patients do live long lives with proper treatments.

We, as oncologists and other specialists, must not have a fatalistic wait-and-see outlook about NETs. This mode of thinking is no longer accurate. We must have knowledge about its possible presence and current treatment options. The cancer survivor must be seen as "a whole person". It is critical to address on-going surveillance, screening and symptom management, from both physical and psychological perspectives.

Although we are more aware today, there is still much work to be done to optimize our educational interventions for survivors and their families, as well as physicians. Now that millions worldwide are living with NETs/carcinoid, it is imperative that among our many priorities we must take a closer look at how we educate our young doctors, other providers, as well as our patients, in order to keep them involved in getting the appropriate care to improve quality of life and prolong lives.

In conclusion, my long career in medical oncology has been rewarding and fulfilling but made more so by being willing to go the extra mile to diagnose and treat complex cancers such as neuroendocrine/carcinoid tumors.

—Phillip Eastman, M.D, Hematologist/Oncologist, Retired

The incidence of carcinoids and neuroendocrine tumors has risen over 500% since 1989 per the SEER Registry kept by the National Cancer Institute. The diagnosis, longitudinal management and care of this rare cancer (approximately 13,000 new cases in the U.S. yearly and prevalence of approximately 160,000) requires dedicated multi-disciplinary centers that include committed surgeons, neuroendocrine and medical oncologists, interventional and nuclear medicine radiologists, gastroenterologists, nutritionists, and mental health professionals. Most importantly, all centers should have a single accountable manager/caregiver for the persons suffering from often times protracted course of NE cancer.

While Europe has developed over 19 centers of excellence in carcinoid and neuroendocrine tumors (sanctioned by the European Neuroendocrine Tumor Society), the U.S., over the past 10 years, has also established several excellent centers for the management and chronic care of this rare cancer. These include:

- *Moffitt Cancer Center, Tampa, Florida (under the direction of Jonathan Strosberg and Larry Kvols)*
- *LSU: Ochsner Medical Center, New Orleans, Louisiana (under the Direction of E.A. Woltering)*
- *Cedars-Sinai, Los Angeles, California (under the direction of Edward Wolin)*
- *East Virginia Medical Center, Norfolk, Virginia (under the direction of A.I. Vinik)*

- *Holden Comprehensive Cancer Center, Iowa City, Iowa (under the co-direction of T.M and M.S. O'Dorisio and James R. Howe)*
- *The Ohio State University (Director, Manisha Shah)*

It is anticipated that with the development of the highly sensitive Ga68-DOTA-modified octreotide-PET Scan and the multi-centered ongoing international LUTATHER Peptide Receptor Radio-Nuclide Therapy (PRRNT), the U.S. will very soon be at parity with our European colleagues who have "forged" and focused the importance and clinical research interest in the management and treatment of neuroendocrine tumors.

Thomas O'Dorisio, M.D
Professor
Endocrine-Metabolism Faculty
Department of Internal Medicine
University of Iowa, Iowa City, Iowa
http://www.int-med.uiowa.edu/divisions/Endocrine/Directory/ThomasO'dorisio.html

Neuroendocrine cancers are an unusual and complicated malignancy that strike people in different ways. Some people can have severe symptoms, some have mild stomach pains, and some may have no problems at all. Regardless of it's presentation, it is imperative to get an early and accurate diagnosis and determine a treatment plan. Unfortunately, since neuroendocrine tumors are rare, most physicians do not have the experience needed to care for them. In these situations, it is important for the patient to be his/her own advocate. Thankfully, there are specialists who purely focus on these diseases and can give you the best advice.

In order to understand why it is important to see neuroendocrine specialists, you have to realize what they can provide for you. The specialist sees many cases of neuroendocrine and has the experience to think beyond what is recommended in the textbooks. Moreover, the specialist is in touch with other specialists who can provide insight into your case. They attend special meetings dedicated to neuroendocrine and hear about the newest findings. They also work closely with physicians in other parts of the world, so if there is a therapy that might be appropriate, but unavailable in the United States, you might still be able to receive it.

The most important part of seeing a neuroendocrine specialist is the fact that they will treat your disease. The art of neuroendocrine is not "what" to do; it is "when" to do it. Neuroendocrine is a different kind of cancer and requires a specialized type of care. It's a team effort that includes the specialist, the local physician, and most importantly the patient. The best care can only be given when the team works well together.

Eric H. Liu, M.D.
Assistant Professor
Department of Surgery, Surgical Oncology
Vanderbilt University Medical Center
(615) 322-2391
www.vanderbiltneuroendocrine.com

Foreword

The standard patient work-up taught in medical schools mandates that all medical students and residents obtain a history and perform a physical examination on all patients. Although physicians and other healthcare providers should never neglect the obvious, emphasis also needs to be placed on going beyond looking for horses if hoof beats are heard, as the symptoms may indicate a zebra. This should become a lifetime practice. The patient's chief complaint or symptoms give clues which will eventually lead to a diagnosis. For example, should the patient present with shortness of breath, the respiratory, circulatory, gastrointestinal, nervous systems, as well as psycho-social status become the main foci for further investigation. Physicians, and other providers who diagnose and treat, are taught to explore signs and symptoms further by talking with the patient, followed by laboratory testing, imaging techniques, and in most cases, obtaining a biopsy. A biopsy is the "gold standard" to prove or disprove a diagnosis such as carcinoma. The combination of the above will eventually lead to a diagnosis.

The problem with neuroendocrine tumors (NETs) is that the symptoms mimic other disease states, because, indeed, these signs and symptoms may be related to "zebras". Sadly, if the provider is not entertaining the possibility of a zebra, the diagnosis is delayed and precious time is lost. One hopes that providers will consider zebras and not just horses, since the most obvious diagnosis may not be correct. Many providers do not "really" listen or may jump to conclusions due to a harried pace in their practice. The patient often leaves the office or hospital with the wrong diagnosis as you will read in the survivor stories. For this reason, the NET community has chosen the zebra as their official mascot. Providers often do not suspect NETs, for they may never see a case in their entire careers. As Susan Anderson says, "If you don't suspect it, you can't detect it".

Neuroendocrine/carcinoid tumors present with a broad spectrum of possible diagnostic signs and symptoms which can be misleading. The possible diagnoses range from irritable bowel syndrome, panic and anxiety attacks, alcoholism, to malingering.

If the patient is a woman, then perimenopause or overt menopause is high on the list of a possible cause for her symptoms. If menopause is ruled out, then anxiety and depression are the second most common diagnoses for women.

NET stands for neuroendocrine tumor; a family of tumors which have certain embryological origins. Carcinoid is in this family and is the most frequent occurring of that group. (Warner, Richard R.P., M.D).

It is estimated that over 90% of persons with NETs are given the wrong diagnosis with treatment rendered for another disease.The average length of time to a correct diagnosis is approximately 7.2 years (Vinik, A.I., MD, et al, 2012). During this time patients often see multiple providers in an effort to find answers while both the disease and it's symptoms continue to worsen. During the process of looking for a diagnosis, and especially if an incorrect one is given, valuable time is lost. Usually, by the time the correct diagnosis of NE cancer is made, metastasis has occurred and cure is no longer an option. Many tumors without symptoms are found during unrelated surgical procedures or at autopsy and are not consistently reported. One wonders how many people have died due to complications of undiagnosed NETs. The key to long term survival is early diagnosis, as approximately 20% of carcinoids are more aggressive than the slow growing ones.

This book is intended to provide information to those with suspicious symptoms which may aid in finding the correct diagnosis so that appropriate testing and treatment will begin as early as possible. The goal is to make this cancer a chronic and controllable disease. There are multiple medical text books, journals, and conferences, all with the common goal of finding an early diagnosis and treatment. This book reminds us that one has to look for "zebras" in the medical workup in order to diagnose NETs. The most often asked questions for both the physician and newly diagnosed will be addressed. The information presented will hopefully aid in reducing the suffering of patients, families and caregivers affected by these tumors.

For those of us living with NETs, it is as though we are dropped off in a barren desert or a jungle and told to find our own way in a bizarre, distorted landscape without a map, much less a compass. There are no landmarks, no signs pointing us towards the correct path (diagnosis).

We are suddenly in a new world where definitions are hard to come by. We live among outlaws: our body's own cells turning mutinous to become silent killers.

We become our own cartographers in order to survive. We grow fluent in medical language which astonishes our family and friends.

We often hear "It's not that bad." "It grows slowly." "We got it all." "You are cured." "You look so good, though". In the meantime, we suffer in silence from the multiple medical problems associated with this cancer.

Our treatments do not often alter our appearance. Therefore carcinoid is often called the "look good cancer". We slide across borders undetected. We live with uncertainty, fear, anxiety and depression. We turn to each other for support and seek out the physicians who have taken an interest in this cancer. Amidst the confusion of managing symptoms with medical, surgical, or radiological interventions, we maintain an attitude of hope.

My desire is that this book will help you come away with a deeper understanding of what NETs are and how people cope with these cancers. The first chapters will serve to educate those who know little if anything about NETs and even those with the disease may find the information of benefit. In the stories, you will learn about the frustration over the seeming lack of knowledge by some of our physicians and the consequences of that ignorance. If our trusted physicians do not look for zebras, to whom do we turn?

Uncertainty does not necessarily need to be feared. It can make one's life bloom—give us power and courage, as you will read in all of the survivors' and caregivers' stories. Self-advocacy emerges, as in "Sunny Susan's" or Lucy Wiley's websites which lend enormous support to the newly diagnosed as well as up-to-date information on the treatments one hopes will continue to emerge. There are several online support groups and social media sites which have become lifelines to information and support. Without them, we would continue to remain lost in the dark!

Medical information is abundant in journals, websites, conferences, through local awareness events, and physicians who have made NETs their specialty. My intent is to inform in a general way versus delving into great detail on the pathophysiology of NE cancer or diverse treatment options which are rapidly evolving.

I appeal to our doctors and other care providers to gain a better understanding of this often "mysterious" cancer and all its manifestations. We often hear "Don't worry, "It is slow growing", "You are lucky, we got it all" or "It is not a type of cancer which could kill you". Many providers still believe that carcinoid, like the word's derivation, is "cancer-like", and not a true cancer. However, this outdated understanding is changing. Carcinoid is a malignant cancer, and, because of its protracted course, those of us who suffer from it are unsung heroes who often have to endure this disease in isolation. As is apparent in the stories that follow, we clearly need earlier diagnosis and treatment.

Those diagnosed with NETs are not in the mainstream. We have no "poster person" for this disease as in breast cancer or HIV disease. The limelight is shed on diseases that are more common, such as myocardial infarctions, strokes, and many others, including other types of cancer.

Our busy medical providers are overwhelmed with caring for acute and chronic illnesses in a largely-broken medical system. One hopes that by shining a light on NE (neuroendocrine cancers), we will achieve greater understanding in the medical field, leading to earlier detection and greater funding for a cure.

There are many unanswered questions about these cancers. Why are there not more clinical trials? Why has it taken 39 years from the time of discovery to treatment with somatostatin analogues? Why are proven treatments and diagnostic tools used in Europe for years not widely available in the United States? These are questions which leave us frustrated and forced to share information with each other which may or may not always be effective but certainly brings us together as a community by design.

This cancer kills and someone is dying because of it as this book is being written and read. My intention is to help raise awareness, perhaps save a life, and empower survivors and caregivers to maintain quality of life by becoming self-advocates.

> *Few doctors in this country seem to be involved with the non-life-threatening side effects of cancer therapy . . . in the United States, baldness, nausea, vomiting, diarrhea, pain, clogged veins, financial problems, broken marriages, disturbed children, loss of libido and self-esteem, as well as body image are nurses' turf . . . It is solely by risking life that freedom is obtained.*

—R. Kushner from The Emperor of All Maladies, S. Mukherjee MD, 2010

A brief overview follows, in an effort to educate those who have never heard of NE cancer. The overview may also help those of us with this disease.

Neuroendocrine & Carcinoid Cancer

Neuroendocrine tumors (NETs) are still considered rare, but recently, there has been an increase in detection due to most medical schools' teaching students to look for rare diseases, as well as better methods of detection. These tumors are typically slow-growing and originate from cells in the endocrine and nervous systems, usually in the gastrointestinal tract. Enterochromaffin cells, give rise to carcinoid tumors. "They were originally identified by a German pathologist in 1907. The term carcinoid means midway between carcinoma and adenoma, a benign growth. Their secretion of serotonin was established in 1953." (ISI, 2013). The most common sites of occurrence are the appendix, ileum, and rectum. Tumors of the small bowel and bronchus have a more malignant course. (Fauci, et al., 2000) Some of the secretions produced by these tumors cause specific syndromes, whereas others are evidenced only by elevations in tumor makers. Sadly, "there is no specific or ideal neuroendocrine tumor marker."

A significant portion of these patients develop symptoms of carcinoid syndrome: flushing, diarrhea or other symptoms such as hemoptysis (blood in sputum) if the tumor originates in the pulmonary system (lungs) valvular heart disease has occurred. The most common hallmark flush associated with carcinoid syndrome occurs in the face and neck area in response to emotions, exercise, drinking alcohol, and eating foods that are high in tyramines. Flushes may be wet or dry. If dry, it is almost always due to a NE tumor. The flush of foregut tumors is long lasting and dry with a purplish or bluish color. The face may develop telangiectasia (broken veins in a spider like distribution). Flushing may be associated with a sensation of warmth and heart palpitations. Tumors of gastrointestinal origin often metastasize to the liver and symptoms may reflect this. NETs may also start out in other organs including the gallbladder, kidneys, liver, lung, ovaries, testis, breast and skeletal system.

NETs behave differently depending on the site of origin or on what unique combination of hormones they secrete. These hormones can cause the symptoms which often are the initial manifestation of the disease. They impact quality of life for those with the disease as one will read in the survivor stories.

The extent of the disease is assessed by lab studies known as biochemical markers, various imaging studies, and watchful waiting for changes in status.

Carcinoid tumors of the gastrointestinal tract, especially those of the small intestine, may be associated with other cancers. These other cancers may be discovered at the same or different times while doctors are investigating signs or symptoms or staging other tumors (Vinik, et al., 2012).

Most NETs of the small and large intestine occur sporadically, while others may occur within the background of an inherited neoplasia syndrome such as multiple endocrine neoplasia type 1 (MEN 1) or (MEN 2). Gastric carcinoids, types 1, 2, and 3, may be associated with chronic atrophic gastritis and other symptoms as well as specific tumor markers. (Vinik, et al., 2012).

As noted, carcinoid is the most common NET. This term will be used often in this book. However the term is slowly being replaced in the medical literature by the term NETs or NE cancer. Neuroendocrine cells receive signals (neurotransmitters released by nerve cells), triggering release of message molecules (hormones) into the circulatory system. The NETs terminology is reflective of the disease's primary origin and the unique characteristics which drive treatment. Some doctors still use the term "carcinoid" when referring to NETs that have developed in the gastrointestinal tract. The terminology can be confusing. For example, a carcinoid may be described as NET or a GEP-NET (gastroenteropancreatic). An insulinoma or islet cell tumor originating in the pancreas may be described as a PET, P-NET, or pancreatic NET (Modlin, 1997).

The intent of this chapter is to give the reader a guide to the terminology surrounding these tumors for a better understanding of the survivors' stories. Also, please refer to the Resource section at the end of this book.

Tumor Characteristics

As noted above, NETs are usually slow-growing ("cancer in slow motion"), as their course of development may take months to years. These tumors are still considered "rare" but recently more cases are diagnosed each year. Treatment for NETs is not always uniform. Different types are managed differently. A patient with NE cancer may have advanced disease by the time of diagnosis, as signs and symptoms are vague and nonspecific.

NET specialists are often located in major cities, and, due to the complexity of this cancer, many patients are still misdiagnosed, especially if they do not have access to care and can't afford to see a specialist. Those in rural areas and of varied ethnic and socio-economic status are at an even greater risk of not being diagnosed until after metastasis has occurred. Therefore, they are seen in the latter stages of the disease when palliation is their only option.

Diagnosis may also be hindered by the nature of some of these tumors. They may remain indolent for years or symptoms may present intermittently. It is not uncommon for an individual with this cancer to be the first to notice symptoms which are compatible with NETs. Often, a person does not seek treatment until tumor burden is such that signs and symptoms began to manifest as pain, weight loss, flushing, or the other symptoms one will read about.

This cancer is a "great masquerader" of many other disease entities, mimicking, for example, anxiety, panic attacks, colitis, Crohn's disease, irritable bowel syndrome, and even varying skin conditions, all which make diagnosis even more complex. Crohn's and irritable bowel syndrome are the two most often diagnosed entities for midgut carcinoids. (www.carcinoid.org).

The diagnosis requires special laboratory and scanning techniques. Many institutions are not familiar with the application of these diagnostic tests and procedures, and may lack specialized equipment. Proper diagnosis mandates specific testing as the diagnosis of neuroendocrine tumors is not a clinical one based solely on symptoms. These special tests may not be available in rural areas, such as Indian reservations or free clinics, thus hindering timely diagnosis.

Biochemical analysis will lead to the diagnosis through identification of the hormones, neuropeptides, and neurotransmitters secreted by these tumors. Imaging studies may show their location and size. These tests also eliminate other disorders that may mimic NETs in the differential diagnosis during the workup of the presenting signs and symptoms.

According to ISI, neuroendocrine cells reside throughout the body in all tissues and can de-differentiate into tumor cells. (ISI, 2013)

Carcinoid Tumors
and Carcinoid Syndrome

As noted, neuroendocrine tumors/neoplasms, are the most commonly occurring gastrointestinal endocrine tumors. The incidence rate is rising. The total age-adjusted incidence rate has increased from 0.62 per 100,000 in 1980 to 5.17 per 100,000 in 2000. (Perez, et al, 2007) The peak incidence of NETs is in the 6th and 7th decade of life but this varies and has been found in children as young as three. (Modlin et al, 2003).

Carcinoid tumors can present in a variety of ways and share certain basic characteristics. Signs and symptoms are vague in the early stages. They may present as intermittent abdominal discomfort or pain, early satiety, bloating, weight loss, overt anorexia, diarrhea and/or flushing. These signs and symptoms may be dismissed by the patient or the health care provider and go undiagnosed for several years or misdiagnosed as another disease entirely.

At least one third of persons with small bowel carcinoid tumors will experience several years of intermittent abdominal pain before being diagnosed. The pain can be due to partial or intermittent obstruction of the bowel. This can lead to the development of intestinal angina, due to bowel ischemia (lack of blood), especially after eating. Kinking of the bowel may also occur and resolve with rest or analgesia (Vinik, A.I., 2010).

If metastasis occurs, it is to regional lymph nodes, liver, and less often to bone, and relates to tumor size. When tumors are discovered at less than 1 cm, the incidence of metastasis is less than 15%. The chances of metastasis increases to 95% with tumors larger than 2 cm. Size alone may not be the only cause for lymphatic or distant spread on an individual basis (Kvols, et al., 2010).

Less Favorable Prognostic Factors for NETs:
Age over 50

- Male gender
- High proliferation index or MIB-1
- Tumor site (pancreas and colorectal)
- Metastases to lymph nodes
- Degree of hepatic metastases (tumor burden)
- Symptomatic mode of discovery
- No surgical curative intent
- Presence of carcinoid syndrome
- Increased chromogranin A, 5-HIAA
- Plasma neuropeptide K (ISI,2013)

The majority of those diagnosed with a NET are already experiencing signs of carcinoid syndrome, but there are exceptions. Some may be asymptomatic until diagnosed. If a tumor is found as an incidental finding during a surgical procedure for some other cause, the chance of a cure rises exponentially.

Carcinoid syndrome is a collection of symptoms that are found in certain individuals with carcinoid tumors. In the most simple cases, this syndrome is associated with midgut carcinoid tumors that have metastasized to the liver. In more complex cases, the syndrome can occur when vasoactive amines such as histamine, serotonin, bradykinin and tachykinin are secreted from the tumor and escape into the systemic circulation. When these amines get into the circulation, they can cause wheezing, flushing, blood pressure changes and diarrhea. Primary tumors of the small bowel and other midgut organs have to be metastatic to have syndrome because the venous outflow of these organs pass through the liver which "filters out" these chemicals before they can escape into the systemic circulation.

—Eugene Woltering, MD, FACS,
LSU Health Sciences Center, New Orleans

Sites Of Tumors

1. Foregut = lung, stomach, pancreas and thymus gland.
2. Midgut = intestine from duodenum to furthest most part of colon.
3. Hindgut = left side of colon and rectum

Rationale for knowing sites of tumors:

Different types are more aggressive than others and respond differently to treatment.

Carcinoid Crisis

Carcinoid crisis [See Appendix III] is the most immediate life-threatening complication of carcinoid syndrome and may occur spontaneously or in response to stress, anesthesia, initiation of chemotherapy, manipulation of involved organs, especially the liver. Carcinoid symptoms that are on-going despite treatment with rescue injections of octreotide need to be treated as an emergency, a true oncologic emergency. Crisis occurs most often in those with foregut tumors with severe symptoms and in those with high urinary 5-HIAA levels. Precautions should be taken with high-risk patients prior to surgical procedures and/or other provoking situations. Octreotide is the drug of choice to treat the crisis.

Symptoms include: generalized flushing and intense diarrhea with abdominal pain as well as cardiac abnormalities with a rapid heart rate (tachycardia) and low blood pressure (hypotension) which can convert to hypertension. There may be ranges of central nervous system deficits from mild light-headedness to loss of consciousness and coma.

Anyone with carcinoid syndrome, who is undergoing any invasive procedure, must decrease the chance of going into full blown crisis by the prophylactic use of octreotide. Prophylaxis is the responsibility of the attending physician and/or the anesthesiologist, usually after being informed by the patient. The risk increases with a larger tumor burden. Carry a card with you that specifies what needs to be done in the event of surgery or other invasive procedures. [See Appendix III] One may schedule an invasive, elective procedure 1-2 weeks after one's IM or SQ (intramuscular or subcutaneous) injection of a somatostatin analog.

Carcinoid Heart Disease

Carcinoid heart disease can develop in those with carcinoid syndrome. The tricuspid or pulmonic valves become thickened due to fibrosis from release of bioactive substances into the hepatic vein by carcinoid liver metastases, leading to right sided heart failure. Tricuspid insufficiency is the predominant finding with tricuspid stenosis (stiffening of the valve). Pulmonary insufficiency and stenosis are less common. Serotonin and bradykinin are implicated in the cause and severity of damage. Findings on echocardiogram or cardiac catheterization will reveal valvular involvement and the need for possible valve replacement. This complication may be on the decrease due to treatment with Sandostatin*, thereby achieving better control of serotonin levels. (Anthony L. and Vinik, AI, 2011).

If cardiac heart disease has occurred, the heart works harder and rhythm disturbances may occur. The patient will experience symptoms of heart failure and pulmonary hypertension.

Symptoms of cardiac involvement include shortness of breath at rest and with exertion, swelling of the lower extremities, need for elevation of the head of the bed with extra pillows in order to sleep (orthopnea), palpitations, pre—or overt syncope (fainting), fatigue, swelling, and possible chest pain.

Medical treatment is necessary to treat the congestive heart failure associated with this condition and includes diuretics to remove retained fluids, as well as medications to strengthen the heart and prevent further decompensation. A note about diuretics: when used to decrease lower extremity edema, some diuretics decrease cardiac output which increases shortness of breath and fatigue. Fluid and sodium are restricted as well. Surgical valve replacement is the only definitive cure. Unfortunately, decreasing urinary 5-HIAA excretions does not reverse cardiac lesions.

Carcinoid Syndrome Triggers-The 5 E's

Carcinoid syndrome can be triggered by any one of the Five "E"'s. Tolerance to each of these seems to be different for each individual.

4. Exercise.
5. Eating certain foods. (Every person has different trigger foods.)
6. Emotion—emotional stress such as anger, fear, depression, grieving and any other emotion in which cortisol, aka adrenaline, is produced in abundance by the adrenal glands.
7. Ethanol—(alcohol), (as little as a few sips).
8. Epinephrine—may be found in analgesics for dental procedures, transdermal patches for pain, as well as in EpiPens® for treatment of allergic reactions. It may also be found in multiple other medical preparations. Always read labels or ask your pharmacist if your medications contain epinephrine. NOTE: Not everyone is affected by epinephrine, as found in Lidoderm patches. Surgery and/or anesthesia can also cause release of epinephrine (adrenalin) (Pommier, R., 2006)

Types of Neuroendocrine Tumors

- PPoma
- PNETs (pancreatic NETs), less than 1 per 100,000 individuals.
- VIPomas (vasoactive intestinal peptide); also called Verner-Morrison syndrome.
- Insulinomas
- Gastrinomas
- Glucagonoma ("Sweet Syndrome")
- Somatostatinoma (SRIF)
- GRFomas (rare)
- Cushing Syndrome
- Goblet Cell tumors
- Pheochromocytomas
- Multiple endocrine neoplasia syndromes, types I and II (MEN-1 and MEN-II)
- Medullary Carcinoma of the Thyroid

- C-Cell Hyperplasia
- Carcinoid (Vinik, et al., ISI, 2013)

Regional Differentiation

Foregut tumors are found in the lungs, stomach, and duodenum. These have a potential for bone metastasis and may be associated with carcinoid syndrome, acromegaly, Cushing's disease, or other endocrine diseases.

Foregut Tumor Biomarker Profile:

- Pancreastatin
- Substance P
- CgA
- 5HIAA

Midgut tumors are the most commonly occurring NE cancers. They are found in the jejunum, ileum, appendix and colon. They are capable of producing high levels of serotonin, kinins, prostaglandins, substance P, and other vasoactive peptides. Bone metastasis can occur, with those located in the jejunum, ileum, and colon, having the greatest potential for metastases to bone. They often metastasize to the liver. (ISI, 2013)

Midgut Tumor Biomarker Profile:

- Neurokinin A (NKA, formerly substance K)
- Pancreastatin
- CgA
- Serotonin
- 5HIAA (serum or urine)

Hindgut tumors are found in the rectum. They rarely produce serotonin or vasoactive peptides. Bone metastasis is not uncommon with these tumors.

Hindgut Tumor Biomarker Profile:

- Pancreastatin
- CgA

Tumors are also classified as functional or non-functional. Functional tumors have a symptomatic course associated with clinical syndromes related to excessive levels of tumor-released bioactive substances. Non-functional tumors are usually not symptomatic. This complicates the diagnostic process due to the lack of neuroendocrine-influenced signs and symptoms and diagnosis is based on exclusion of diseases which masquerade as NETs (Vinik et al, 2012)

Some Clinical Manifestations of NETs

Intestinal Carcinoid

- Abdominal pain
- Bowel obstruction
- Flushing
- Fatigue
- Weight loss
- Bloating
- Early satiety
- Diarrhea

Bronchial Carcinoid

- Wheezing with bronchoconstriction
- Cough with possible chest pain
- Bloody sputum
- Bronchospasm—may be associated with flushing episodes and cannot be treated as an asthma attack, due to use of epinephrine which provokes a vasomotor response that may result in death. Steroids are the preferred treatment.

Pancreatic NETs

- Epigastric pain
- Chronic peptic ulcer disease

- Intermittent low blood sugar levels
- Rash/dermatitis
- Diabetes
- Diarrhea
- Weight loss

Other

- Right valvular heart disease; (see cardiac manifestations) Excessive levels of serotonin cause scarring of the tricuspid valve.
- Changes in skin pigmentation, usually hyperpigmentation
- Muscle and joint pain (chronic pain syndrome)
- Poor absorption of nutrients, especially if intestinal resection has been done. Fat soluble vitamins may be poorly absorbed, as well as essential minerals and oils such as essential fatty acids which the body does not make and must therefore be exogenous (taken as a supplement) (NIH, 2012)

Common Amines and Peptides, produced by NETs which cause symptoms

(50 have been identified; 6 listed)

- Serotonin
- Histamine
- Substance P
- Tachykinins
- Kallikrein
- Prostaglandins (Anthony, B. Lowell, MD, 2004)

The most important take away message from the above information is that any person presenting with irritable bowel syndrome or other symptoms such as abdominal pain, flushing, or unexplained weight loss that may mimic carcinoid syndrome must be evaluated for neuroendocrine cancer. It is better to be safe than sorry and one may need to advocate for this evaluation!

Imaging for Diagnosing NETs

- Ultrasound
- CT—Multi-phasic with contrast (unless allergic)
- MRI
- PET Scan
- OctreoScan™ with SPECT
- Angiography
- Gallium-68 (Ga^{68}) DOTA PET
- Endoscopy
- Capsule Endoscopy
- Double Balloon Endoscopy
- Emerging imaging procedures (Liu,E. 2013 UCSF Conference.)
- Chest x-ray, CT or if necessary, bronchoscopy
- Echocardiogram (to evaluate for cardiac heart disease, especially if metastasis has occurred, regardless of symptoms of carcinoid syndrome at presentation).

Treatment of NETs

- Surgical Resection or debulking of tumors.
- Somatostatin analogs such as Sandostatin LAR* or Lanreotide Depot* (somatuline), octreotide (generic)
- Afinitor* or other chemotherapeutic agents
- Chemoembolization
- HACE (Hepatic Artery Chemoembolization)
- SIR Spheres*
- Thera-Spheres*
- Targeted radiation
- Conventional Chemotherapy
- RFA (Radio-frequency Ablation)
- VEGF pathway inhibitors (mTor inhibitors)
- Nanoknife* or cryo-knife
- PRRNT (PRRT) (Peptide Receptor Radionuclide Therapy)
- Clinical trials (Kulke,2003, Fisher, G., 2013)
- New and emerging treatments

Prognosis

Every person has a unique prognosis and needs to be managed individually. The presentation may be different, thus the treatment of these changes should be addressed on an individual basis. Diligence in monitoring disease progression is essential to prevent complications which may affect one's outcome.

Prognosis and treatment options vary widely. For the common mid-gut carcinoid patient, prognosis depends on location of the tumor, pathology results, the size and type of the tumor. Smaller tumors are less likely to have already metastasized or spread regionally to more distant areas such as vital organs. Once liver metastasis has occurred, prognosis becomes less favorable. Carcinoid syndrome or cardiac involvement may already be a factor. Prognosis also depends on whether the tumor can be completely excised and whether the presentation of the cancer is newly diagnosed or a recurrence.

Another consideration is overall health status, as well as co-morbidities such as diabetes, coronary artery disease, and immune disorders. These all impact prognosis. Medications that suppress the immune system, such as long-term steroid use, also adversely affect outcome. A person's psycho-social status can impact survival. Good family or community support, monetary stability and a good outlook on life are critical assets for a favorable prognosis.

For additional resources on evolving diagnostic, monitoring, and treatments, refer to the websites listed in the Resource chapter.

Monitoring NETs and Disease Progression

Pathology

Analysis of tissue removed during biopsy or surgical removal of an organ, is used for staging and evaluation of disease status. This important tool helps to evaluate disease status.

Some of the tests specific to NETs are listed below.

- **Chromogranin A (CgA)**—a biomarker; the precursor to several functional peptides including vasostatin, pancreastatin, and parastatin. This test is used for prognosis and follow-up. Note that increase in CgA levels is not limited to carcinoid tumors.

- **Ki-67**—a protein cellular marker that shows how fast cancer cells multiply. This is probably the most important marker for predicting overall survival.
- **P-53**—a tumor suppressor protein.
- **C-Kit**—a protein on the surface of some cells, found at high levels or in a changed form on some types of cancer cells.
- **Mitotic count**—measures the rate of cell growth. The more cells that are dividing, the more aggressive the cancer.

Monitoring

NETs, as with any cancer or illness, needs to be monitored on a regular basis. This may vary according to type of NET, one's oncologist and insurance coverage. The usual interval for blood analysis of biomarkers, complete blood count (CBC with differential), liver panel, especially if there is metastasis to the liver, is every three to six months once stability has been achieved. Other tests are at the discretion of the provider and may be driven by change in status which may indicate disease progression. This holds true for diagnostic imaging, which may also be required before and after interventions.

The most common tests for the common mid-gut carcinoid patient include serotonin levels, chromogranin A, 5-HIAA, pancreastatin, neurokinin A, and substance P.

Echocardiograms should be done at the time of diagnosis as a baseline and yearly thereafter.

This ultrasound is done more frequently if a person begins to exhibit signs and symptoms of heart valve involvement which is attributed to the release of large amounts of serotonin. This will be evident by signs and symptoms of heart failure. In addition, visits to one's oncologist should occur routinely every four to six months, or more often, as mandated by the disease process and patient status. (Warner, A., 2002).

Biomarkers

5-HIAA—a metabolite of serotonin. This test measures the breakdown of serotonin by the liver and is a 24—hour urine collection. Blood assay is now available.

Test results of the urinary 5-HIAA can be elevated by the consumption of certain foods (can cause false positive readings), and should be avoided for 48 hours prior to the collection of the urine sample. Note: keep urine in refrigerator until collection is complete. The foods to avoid include caffeine, avocados, bananas, tomatoes, plums, walnuts, pineapple, eggplant, kiwi, plantains, as well as nicotine, red wine, cheese, hot dogs, chocolate, vanilla containing foods, custard, cassava, hickory, and pecans.

Drugs that can decrease urinary levels include heparin, isoniazid (INH), levodopa, MAO inhibitors, methenamine, levodopa, phenothiazines such as Compazine*, tricyclic anti-depressants, reserpine, methocarbamol, glyceryl (found in many cough preparations, phenacetin, Tylenol, salicylates.(ISI, 2013)

Serum Serotonin—or 5-HT, is a monoamine neurotransmitter. This test measures serotonin levels in the blood. Serotonin is the most common hormone of carcinoid cancer. Elevated levels can cause carcinoid syndrome. Serotonin occurs naturally in the body and is responsible for gut motility in the gastric system. It is also responsible for regulation of mood, appetite, and sleep. The food restrictions for the urinary test for serotonin do not apply to this blood analysis. An overnight fast is required, however. (ISI, 2013)

Chromogranin A—May be the most stable of tests for disease progression and may play a role in early neoplastic (new growth) progression. Ascitic fluid CgA may be measured if ascites develops. This test hould be done in a fasting state and after stopping PPI's or H2 blockers (antacid medications) for seven to ten days.

Neurokinin A (formerly known as substance K)—is a member of the tachykinin family of neuropeptide neurotransmitters and has been shown to have a strong prognostic value. Any alteration in NKA predicts improved or worsening survival.

Pain medications, anti-hypertensives, and medications that affect gastrointestinal function should be avoided for forty eight hours prior to testing. (ISI, 2013)

Pancreastatin—A rapid rise in levels of this marker while on somatostatin analogue therapy is associated with poor survival in well differentiated NET patients. Pancreastatin tends to rise earlier than

Chromogranin A. This blood test is useful for monitoring treatment response as well.

- **Pancreatic primary**: nonspecific markers (Chromogranin A, pancreatic polypeptide, substance P) and specific markers depending on clinical signs and symptoms. Markers may include 5-HIAA /serotonin, gastrin, glucagon, insulin, VIP (vasoactive intestinal polypeptide).
- **Lung primary**: Chromogranin A, neuron specific enolase (NSE), 5-HIAA / serotonin, substance P, ACTH.
- **Intestinal primary**: Chromogranin A, substance P, 5-HiAA, Serotonin, substance P, urinary methyl-histamine (gastric primaries only).
- **Rectal primaries**: usually have NO elevated markers.
- **Carcinoid**: CgA, pancreastatin, neurokinin A, substance P, 5-HIAA (24 hour urine)
- **Unknown primary:** Chromogranin A, 5-HIAA / serotonin, NSE, substance P (Vinik et al., 2013)

Imaging and Recommendations for Follow-up

CT/MRI—every six to twelve months, or at the discretion of one's physician and change in status.

(Note that MRI is the preferred imaging modality for monitoring liver metastases).

OctreoScan™—baseline and if indicated by clinical or radiographic changes.

Ga[68] DOTA-TATE PET scan—This diagnostic imaging study has a much higher sensitivity than the OctreoScan™, and therefore can detect more and smaller tumors than conventional CT, MRI, or OctreoScan™. While available in Europe, India, Israel and other countries outside the United States, at the time of publication, only a few institutions in the U.S. offer this scan (Vanderbilt University and the University of Iowa), but many instituitions are preparing to do so.

Echocardiogram—baseline and yearly for functioning carcinoid patients. This ultrasound becomes more important in those with high serotonin levels because of the risk of valvular heart disease.

Bone Densitometry (DEXA)
The preservation of bone mass can be affected by immobility brought on by pain, fatigue, depression, malabsorption of nutrients such as vitamin D and calcium due to diarrhea, treatment with steroids and avoidance or inability to bear weight or exercise.

Quality of Life Issues for NET Patients

As with any cancer or life-threatening illness, quality of life (QOL) becomes one of the most important concerns for all involved. The phase that follows the initial diagnosis of any cancer is complex and individual. It can offer components of healing, re-awakening and discovery of a new life. Because of the possibility of prolonged survival in NETs, quality of life is a high priority. The most prevalent concerns for NET survivors include incapacitating symptoms such as diarrhea, fatigue, pain, and weight loss. Worry about illness progression, generalized anxiety and depression also impinge QOL.

All issues surrounding a diagnosis of a life threatening illness are colored by frustration, ongoing fear and worries about finances. There is also the issue of the impact of the stigma of cancer, especially one as complex and misunderstood as neuroendocrine cancer. Most persons with NETs do not appear ill; therefore, it is difficult to convey that one has cancer. Many with this cancer are met with skepticism due to their "look good" appearance.

The bodily changes in NETs are not as prevalent as in other types of rapidly growing or disfiguring cancers. In fact, the great majority of persons with NETs appear healthy until the late stages of the disease. NET patients report worse QOL than the general population in several studies conducted in multiple countries. An on-line survey revealed that general health scores were significantly associated with the type of NET, current presence of tumor, carcinoid syndrome, and frequency of bowel movements. (Pancreas, Vol.39, #6, August, 2010).

"It's hard work behaving as a credible patient"
—Melanie Thernstrom

"My People are destroyed for lack of knowledge."

Hosea 4:6

Improving Quality of Life

While somatostatin analogues have improved quality of life for those with diarrhea, there are many other issues that need addressing to improve coping skills.

When done on a regular basis, exercise helps by improving the immune system's ability to fight disease, including cancer. It also gives one a sense of well-being due to the expression of endorphins, the body's natural morphine. Exercise also lowers levels of several key blood-borne markers of chronic inflammation (C-reactive protein or CRP). In addition, homocysteine levels, another marker of inflammation, are lowered within at least 30 minutes of aerobic exercise three times a week. This exercise regimen can be broken up into three ten minute intervals a day. Strength training with resistance bands or light weights builds muscle mass which may prevent falls.

Exercise helps us adapt to stress by preventing abnormal stress-induced cortisol secretion. It can reverse insulin resistance, especially for those on somatostatin analogues, which can cause hypoglycemia or hyperglycemia. High levels of cortisol and glucose in our bloodstream harm our immune system. One can begin a walking program for at least 30 minutes a day. If one is unable to walk for thirty minutes, start with five or ten minutes and work one's way up as tolerated. (AARP, July/August 2007; 30-32) (Alschuler & Gazella, 2011)

Most persons with carcinoid may have carcinoid syndrome triggered by exercise. Therefore, it is recommended that exercise be carried out as tolerated. A pre-exercise octreotide injection may be necessary to offset symptoms such as flushing.

Proper nutrition ranks high on the list of therapeutic factors by providing the nutrients one needs to maintain health and replace lost calories or electrolytes. Shared meals also provide a social event which gives us a sense of wellbeing. When foods we once loved and shared with others contribute to symptoms, this becomes a void that is difficult to fill. That special food or meal becomes yet one more roadblock impacting quality of life and may be hard for family and friends to understand. With patience and teaching, relatives and friends will be more than willing to adapt to changes to prevent problems for their loved ones.

The most important thing to focus on is eating a healthy, balanced diet when one is feeling well. If appetite is poor, eat what is appealing and well-tolerated. The goal is to maintain weight during treatment.

Plan activities when one is most alert. Pain medications may prevent one from being fully present until dosing is adequate to render a pain free state without grogginess. Opiates may also cause anorexia.

Suitable activities should not rob one of energy. One may need to change activities of daily living by incorporating the help of others or use of aids such as sitting on a stool when prepping meals. That which is enjoyable should add to quality of life and not be a hindrance. The body will let one know about limitations which may change from day to day.

Let others help you! When friends offer to help, let yourself be loved. Feel good about taking their offers and have a task in mind for your support system. Let go of things that don't bring you joy or cause distress. Getting eight to ten hours of sleep on a consistent basis is recommended as well as one to two naps per day to enhance healing and offset the impact of stress.

Conquer pain. Speak with your doctor about pain. Be specific about location, quality, and times of day when it is most prevalent. Use a pain scale to describe pain. The usual pain scale is numerical, with "1" indicating pain that is a minor annoyance and "10" the most severe. Discuss side effects of pain medications. Keep a pain log to track changes over time.

Seek out anything that brings pleasure! As Norman Cousins so well demonstrated, "laughter is the best medicine." Therefore, go beyond staying positive and seek out humor in life. There are laughter clinics as therapy available in many cities.

Friends, family, and pets can surround us with love. Friends and family can listen to our concerns, run errands, clean our homes, or shop and prepare meals. Be creative and allow friends and family to help. The American Cancer Society offers rides to patients to and from medical appointments.

Spirituality or religion offer comfort and lead to the release of endorphins which in turn lead to a quiet mind and relieve fear.

Meditation or anything that quiets the mind will also help with a sense of control of negative emotions which can be detrimental to mental and physical health.

Therapy and support groups enhance QOL by helping to let go of issues that impede healing. A sense of camaraderie is, in itself, healing.

Use a financial counselor to help work through changes in income and estate planning.

Enlist the aid of social workers, clergy, and ombudsman from your insurance plan in a hospital or clinic.

Always carry information about your disease:

- The protocol for treatment of carcinoid crisis
- All relevant current medications
- Allergies
- People to notify in case of emergencies
- A copy of your durable power of attorney
- A list of prior surgeries, treatments

Alert all care providers (e.g. dentists) about the risk for carcinoid crisis. Wear a Medic Alert bracelet that informs others that you have carcinoid or other neuroendocrine cancers. You may choose to carry syringes and some octreotide in a cooling pack with you for medical procedures.

Arrive at medical appointments with questions for your medical provider. Ask for explanations of anything you do not understand. Be organized, stay focused on the disease, set the tone, be understanding and compassionate of your provider's possible lack of knowledge and time limitations.

Choose a provider who is open to learning about your cancer. Never be afraid of your doctor. You have hired a health care provider to assist you and therefore have the right to communicate with him or her. You have the right to ask for and receive as many opinions as you want. You have the right to terminate your relationship with a health care provider as well. You also have the right to appeal a denied diagnostic test or treatments.

At the time of this writing, continued assessment of QOL in future longitudinal studies and clinical trials will help identify and confirm what really impacts NET patient's QOL in order to provide better disease management. In the meantime you have the ability to focus on your quality of life and take actions to improve it.

Quality of Life: Details

NET patients face many challenges in the course of their disease due to the side effects of treatment, medications, the stress of the disease itself, fear of progression and the myriad issues associated with this cancer.

What follows is a synopsis of some of the issues we face on a daily basis and how to approach them for better outcomes.

Malabsorption

Prolonged diarrhea is usually associated with weight loss, and the specific causes of the resulting malabsorption are usually established based on physiological evaluations. Anyone experiencing protracted diarrhea should seek the care of a doctor to rule out malabsorption. The treatment depends on the cause and type of malabsorption.

Your doctor may do a medical workup to rule out celiac disease, an immunoglobulin A (IgA) deficiency, and/or order stool studies to try to distinguish between parasitic or other intestinal causes if you are diagnosed with malabsorption. NE cancer can produce diarrhea, leading to malabsorption, depending on what specific hormones are released by an individual's tumors.

In cases of severe intestinal disease, such as extensive regional enteritis (requiring, for example, large resection or a total gastrectomy), then total parenteral nutrition (TPN) may become necessary. This is usually a treatment that is employed to rest the bowel and /or maintain a person's nutritional state until further treatment can be carried out. It may also be used if a person can no longer eat. TPN can have inherent problems, such as sepsis, if the catheter site into the body becomes infected or for other reasons/causes.

Examples of the work-up for the cause of diarrhea:

- Small bowel series using barium. CT scan of the abdomen to detect possible evidence of chronic pancreatitis, enlarged lymph nodes as seen in lymphoma or Whipple disease.

- Endoscopic retrograde cholangiography and pancreatography (ERCP): this study helps document malabsorption due to pancreatic or biliary-related disorders.
- Plain abdominal x-ray (flat and upright): pancreatic calcifications are indicative of chronic pancreatitis as are pseudo cysts. This series can also reveal air fluid levels, indicative of a bowel obstruction.
- Shilling test: for malabsorption of vitamin B_{12}, especially in gastric resection, bacterial overgrowth, ileal resection or disease. Note: this test is rarely done these days as there are more sophisticated methods assessing B_{12} malabsorption.
- Stool for culture and to rule out ova and parasites.
- Upper endoscopy with small bowel mucosal biopsies from different sites of the bowel to establish a definitive diagnosis of malabsorption. This should be determined by your physician.
- Colonoscopy may also be of use. For example, it may uncover autoimmune colitis, or other diseases of the bowel.

Abdominal Distension

Bacterial fermentation of unabsorbed food substances releases gaseous products such as hydrogen and methane, causing flatulence (gas). Flatulence often causes uncomfortable abdominal distention and cramps.

Relief may be found by using over the counter medications that are simethicone based. It is wise to avoid gas producing foods or take Beano* with the first bite of foods known to be gas producers, such as beans and others legumes as well as cruciferous (cabbage family) vegetables. Before cooking, soaking beans until they just begin to sprout, changing the water twice a day, will facilitate digestion.

There are products on the market such as "Subtle Butt" that are disposable gas neutralizers which contain activated carbon. They are worn inside the under garments, as a liner, and can be effective for social events. For more information, see: www.solutionsthatstick.com.

A more serious form of abdominal distension is found in liver failure. This is an accumulation of fluid in the peritoneal cavity known as ascites. Small amounts may be asymptomatic, while increasing amounts cause abdominal distension and discomfort, anorexia, nausea, early satiety, heartburn, flank pain, and respiratory distress due to pressure on the diaphragm from an enlarging abdomen. Treatment is palliative and includes paracentesis, a drawing out of fluids with a needle. This procedure is done for comfort and can be repeated as needed. Medications are given to help manage portal hypertension which may accompany liver failure.

Abdominal distension also occurs with a partial or complete obstruction of the bowel. Obstructions may be caused by adhesions from prior surgery, bowel kinking, tumor growth and it's associated ischemia or desmoplastic response to cancer in general. While adhesions are the most prominent cause of small bowel obstruction, approximately 40% of obstructions occur in patients who have never had a surgical procedure. (Shelton, 1999)

Early symptoms of a bowel obstruction may include intermittent cramping, overt abdominal pain that is constant and increases in severity, constipation or a sense of inability to evacuate the bowel completely, inability to pass gas, bloating, nausea, vomiting, and high pitched, loud sounds from the intestines (borborygmi). These symptoms mandate a visit to an Emergency Department for treatment with a nasogastric tube to keep the gut decompressed and rest the bowel. If the obstruction is not relieved by these conservative measures, which also include nothing by mouth and intravenous hydration, surgery is an option to determine what is causing the obstruction.

Edema

Edema is soft tissue swelling due to abnormal expansion of interstitial fluid volume. It can be limited to a particular organ or vascular bed. Unilateral extremity edema is usually due to venous or lymphatic obstruction as found in tumor obstruction. Ascites may also be present as isolated and localized edema due to inflammation or neoplasm.

One can also have generalized edema in which soft tissue swelling of most or all areas of the body occur. Ascites and edema of the lower extremities and scrotum are frequent in cirrhosis or congestive heart failure. Edema may also occur with kidney disease or may be idiopathic (cause unknown). Hypothyroidism, caused by use of somatostatin analogs or an autoimmune disorder can also cause edema which is typically located in the lower extremities or around the eyes (periorbital) and is corrected by replacement of thyroid hormone. Other causes of edema include drugs such as steroids, estrogens, and vasodilators such as amlodipine (Norvasc'). There are others that are beyond the scope of this book.

A low albumin level, from chronic protein malabsorption or from losses of protein into the intestinal lumen, causes edema of the lower extremities. With severe protein depletion, ascites may also develop.

In summary, treatment of edema due to multiple causes is aimed at the cause and can include paracentesis, salt and fluid restriction, elastic (TED) hose, elevation of the lower extremities, diuretics and other medications to manage symptoms and help with palliation.

Anemia

Anemia is defined as the body not having enough red cells to carry adequate oxygen to all parts of the body. The definition of anemia can also be viewed as: blood hemoglobin (Hb) concentration, less than 140 grams per liter (less than 14 grams/dL, or hematocrit (Hct), less than 42 % in adult males; Hb less than 120 grams/liter (less than 12 grams/dL) or Hct less than 37% in adult females. Anemias are classified as microcytic (small red cells, as in iron deficiency), or macrocytic (large cells, as in B_{12} deficiency). Other disease states may cause anemia. Your doctor will evaluate the cause.

Ileal involvement such as ileal resection can cause megaloblastic anemia due to vitamin B_{12} deficiency.

If Vitamin K is not absorbed, this can lead to bleeding disorders, easy bruising, or even blood in the stool which manifests as dark, black (tarry) stools, or blood in the urine (hematuria).

Anemia is treated by iron replacement or blood transfusions followed by correction of the cause.

Complete iron studies should be assessed with a diagnosis of anemia: Iron and saturation levels, total iron binding capacity (TIBC), and ferritin levels. A complete blood count (CBC with differential) tracks the treatment's efficacy.

If anemia is recalcitrant to treatment, more sophisticated testing is necessary, such as bone marrow aspiration for further analysis of the cause (may need to rule out leukemia or other disease states such as chronic kidney disease; nephrotic syndrome).

Metabolic Defects of Bones

Vitamin D deficiency can cause bone disorders such as osteopenia or osteomalacia. If not corrected, osteopenia can lead to overt osteoporosis. This can lead to spontaneous fractures of the long bones of the body, bone pain, or vertebral body collapse. Treatment is medical or surgical to prevent destruction; you and your physician will decide the best course of action. Metastases to bone must always be ruled out with new or changing bone pain.

Vitamin C is crucial to shaping and growing bones. We know the importance of calcium for bone health, but calcium in a vacuum is ineffective. Vitamin C increases the solubility of calcium. After taking a calcium supplement, the body works to dissolve it in the stomach. Increased solution means increased absorption so more can actually get to your bones. Anything that aids in the process is very helpful, as our ability to dissolve capsules, tablets and food diminishes as we grow older, due to the weakening of stomach acid. High levels of calcium in the body can contribute to low stomach acid; therefore, taking Vitamin C can support a more healthy digestive process. (Dewey, M., 2013)

The recommended intake for Vitamin C is 75 mg. for adult females and 90 mg. for adult males. (U.S. Food and Nutrition Board of the Institute of Medicine).

Malabsorption of calcium can lead to secondary hyperparathyroidism, characterized by elevated serum calcium, constipation, depression, peptic ulcer disease, bone pain, fatigue, anorexia, nausea, and in late stages, mental status changes and other abnormalities in blood work (abnormal parathyroid hormone level). It is a generalized disorder of bone metabolism due to increased secretion of parathyroid hormone by an adenoma or carcinoma. Familial hyperparathyroidism may be part of multiple endocrine neoplasia Type 1 (MEN1), which also includes pituitary and pancreatic tumors as well as hypergastrinemia with peptic ulcer disease (Zollinger-Ellison Syndrome). Hyperparathyroidism may occur in NETs, diagnosed by patient history and biochemical analysis. Hyperparathyroidism can affect bone. It is confirmed by demonstration of an inappropriately high PTH level as well as a high calcium and albumin. Hypercalcemia (high calcium levels in the blood) is a dangerous situation that will need immediate attention by your physician. (Adler, M.D., 2013).

Neurological Manifestations

Electrolyte disturbances such as hypocalcemia (low calcium), and hypomagnesemia (low magnesium), can lead to tetany, an involuntary contraction of muscles.

Vitamin malabsorption can cause generalized motor weakness (pantothenic acid, vitamin D) or peripheral neuropathy (thiamine and other B vitamins), loss of vibratory sensation and position (cobalamin), night blindness (vitamin A), and seizures (biotin). Hair loss is also attributed to malabsorption of these vitamins.

In summary, NETs can deplete the body of important vitamins and minerals when diarrhea and malabsorption are untreated. By judiciously adding these to one's diet, preferably under medical supervision, complications can be resolved.

Pain

We will all have pain at some point in our lives. With a diagnosis of neuroendocrine cancer, and possible resultant surgery, we will most certainly face pain. Pain in NETs is common even without surgery and may be the first clue we get that our body is not in homeostasis (stable equilibrium).

Pain from NETs can become chronic and unrelenting. Not all pain is neuropathic. It can be muscular, post-surgical, inflammatory, or psychogenic (physical pain that is caused, augmented, or prolonged by emotional factors). Conditions causing pain usually cause multiple types of pain. However, many chronic pain complaints have a hidden neuropathic component. Over time, neuropathic pain leads to musculoskeletal pain. Nerve pain creates muscle spasms which in turn interfere with normal use of the affected area. This can lead to weakness, immobility, and eventually atrophy and contractures. These changes can lead to mood disorders and insomnia, and the original problem becomes more difficult to detect. In NETs, with multiple types of affectations, pain becomes more difficult to define and treat. These problems are often misdiagnosed, widespread and undertreated.

(Thernstrom, M., 2010)

Many with NETs produce hormones which cause inflammation which leads to pain, both acute and chronic. Other causes of pain may include: inflammation of joints, recovery from surgery, tumor growth, or neuropathies.

Recent research shows that pain produces pathological changes in the brain and spinal cord. Unfortunately, many patients and doctors still have misguided beliefs and outdated dogmas that prevent proper treatment. This can have devastating effects on quality of life.

Many in pain are treated as drug seekers or hypochondriacs and suffer the consequences. Chronic pain can lead to depression and depression can lead to more pain, a vicious cycle that is hard to break. (Thernstrom, M., 2010)

It is not uncommon for pain to be improperly evaluated and controlled. Our doctors or other providers may seem oblivious to the severity of our pain. Most of us avoid returning to our doctors for fear of reprisal, or we accept their pain medication as the only way to cope with our pain.

In the last few years, pain treatment has emerged as a separate entity, with pain clinics and pain specialists now available. These clinics offer multiple means to treat pain. At the forefront are opioids and muscle relaxants. Opioids are a mainstay for chronic pain management!

Chronic opioid therapy (COT) may be considered if chronic pain is moderate or severe, has an adverse impact on function or quality of life, and the potential benefits outweigh the potential harm. A benefit to harm evaluation should be performed.

Ongoing discussion with you, the patient, regarding COT, should be performed.

Many doctors are now obtaining consent for treatment with opioids. Random urine testing has also come into play lately, due to abuse by those who are not using these drugs for pain. Sadly, this is a barrier for us when we need pain medications, but with a team approach, we and our oncologists can tailor an effective individualized treatment plan.

- Never take someone else's pain medications.
- Never adjust your own dose.
- Never mix with alcohol.
- Do not take with antidepressants, sleep aids or anti-anxiety medications.
- Always keep your medications locked in a safe place.

Free patient education materials
are available from a number of sources, e.g.:
www.painAction.com
and
www.er-la-opioidrems.com/IwgUI/rems/ped.action.
(Pri-Med Webinar, 2013.

Acupuncture has emerged as a vital and credible means to address pain. Massage, moxibustion, heat, ice, relaxation, meditation, medical cannabis, and guided visualization are also employed in pain management.

A pain diary is recommended so that you and your provider can determine if your pain is being treated adequately. Adjustments to your pain control regimen can then be made.

Much can be said about pain, an experience one is never in doubt about having. Pain can also be classified as an emotion. One can have mental pain without physical pain, especially with cancer. In our Western world we view mental and physical pain as separate entities, but fortunately this is changing. Therefore, pain's complex relationship with the person experiencing it is as unique as our emotions.

All of us who suffer pain of any kind need not feel alone or untreated. A basic human right is to alleviate suffering and we, together with advocates, can do much to prevent needless and detrimental suffering. (Thernstrom, 2010).

Nutrition

With a diagnosis of cancer, optimal nutrition is an integral part of improving the body's immune function and controlling symptoms. Consuming a healthy, balanced diet is best but often not feasible for various reasons. Many people with cancer often lack the appetite necessary to take in an adequate number of calories or eat foods which will supply the necessary nutrients needed by the body for repair. Depression may also play a role in a person's ability to ingest an adequate amount of calories. Diarrhea in NETs is the biggest fear for many when it comes to eating. A state of nutritional deficiency then ensues.

When a person has cancer, there is a need for extra protein to help in the healing process which is altered due to the cancer itself, chemotherapy, or other medications. (Alschuler, L, ND, 2011). The body's chemistry needs to be made less acidic and more alkaline. Cancer cells thrive in a highly acidic environment. Daily consumption of deep green leafy vegetables such as collard greens, kale, Swiss chard, turnip greens, is vital.

One needs to consume 60-70 grams (1.5 grams per kilogram of body weight) of protein a day to maintain healthy bones and muscles, says Leslie Bonci, M.P.H., R.D., at the University of Pittsburgh Medical Center. If one is unable to consume this amount by eating whole foods, supplements may provide the necessary amount needed. Fats, fiber, and sugar are not recommended in persons with NETs. Cancer is an urgent call to stop eating animal protein as well as the foods mentioned below. (Emeka, M. L., Cancer's Best Medicine)

"Niacin deficiency, general protein energy deficiency, nutrition problems due to surgery, malnutrition and chronic diarrhea, and the excess metabolism of tryptophan," are the key nutritional issues for carcinoid patients, says endocrinologist Jeffrey I. Mechanick, M.D.

A high protein diet is high in tryptophan. It is estimated that more than 60% of tryptophan in our bodies is taken in by tumors for synthesis of serotonin. Tryptophan is also necessary for the synthesis of other proteins and niacin (B_3). The medications that many NET patients take to control symptoms often bring on hyperglycemia, so there is a benefit to staying lean. (Alschuler, et al., 2011).

MCT (medium chain triglycerides) oil is also recommended to maintain lean body mass. One is advised to check with a nutritionist and your physician before taking this oil.

Phytochemicals help the liver with its detoxification process. Examples of phytochemicals include: green tea without milk as milk renders the tea less beneficial. Other examples include cold-water fatty fish such as salmon, supplemental Vitamin D3 to maintain a level close to 50-60 (serum levels which should be checked at least every three months). (Macaire, G., RD, UCSF, 2013.)

Persons with NETs are prone to multiple nutrient deficiencies due to the disease process itself or surgical interventions that may contribute to short gut syndrome, especially in midgut carcinoids. Malabsorption needs to be ruled out. The type will be determined by your physician, but most is secretory in nature. Small bowel surgery can impede absorption of fat soluble vitamins and other nutrients, such as B_{12} and most of the B vitamins which are essential for hair and nail growth, health of nerves, and the nervous system in general.

Note that opiates have an adverse effect on bones and can lead to osteopenia and osteoporosis.

"Most cancer patients don't die from their tumors—they die of malnutrition, toxemia, and/or infections. Proper nutrition can help address all of these."
                                    —Susan Silberstein, PhD (Hungry for Health)

Poor Appetite / Nausea / Vomiting

Some tips for handling the most prevalent side effects of cancer and its treatment:

Eat small meals that appeal to you, and eat them often—four to six times a day is recommended.

Drink fluids between meals to avoid feeling "full" at meal time. Avoid drinking water with meals, as it dilutes necessary enzymes and stomach acid, unless oral sores or difficulty in swallowing are problematic.

Keep saltine crackers (contraindicated by a low-sodium diet) and sparkling water handy for times when you feel especially nauseated.

Graze throughout the day so you always have food in your stomach.

Often times, warm foods such as tea, soups, warm milk (unless lactose intolerant), almond, rice or soy milk, yogurt, sorbet or a low fat milk shake can be appealing.

Smoothies made with added protein powder and fruits that are tolerable to you are also recommended. (Note: if you are receiving oxaliplatin chemotherapy, avoid cold foods).

For main meals and snacks: white toast, white rice, potatoes, boiled and without the skin, pasta or noodles, oatmeal, crackers, pretzels, cream of wheat or rice, broiled or baked chicken without the skin unless one is vegetarian.

Some people find that ginger helps with nausea. Ginger intake may be in the form of slices of raw ginger root, tea, ale, or sugarless candy.

Weight Loss

If weight loss occurs, eat small, frequent meals throughout the day (5-6 times or every 3-4 hours).

Try eating foods high in calories such as natural peanut or other nut butters, eggs, yogurt, nuts, avocado and soups to boost your intake. This is a time when the fat content of food should not be of concern unless fat causes diarrhea, which can be ameliorated by enzymes such as Creon˚.

Use sauces, dips, cheeses and whole fat dairy products (unless you are lactose intolerant) to help boost calories. Add skim milk powder to food to increase protein value as well.

Nutritional drinks or other shakes can help you get the nutrition you need when you are not able to eat very much. I recommend Peptamen® or Glucerna® as they are low in sugar and Peptamen® contains probiotics which help the immune system, especially if diarrhea is a problem. Probiotics replace good bacteria in the gut, thus maintaining the normal flora. Begin slowly with probiotics as they can lead to gas and bloating.

Enteric coated peppermint may help relieve these symptoms: abdominal pain, diarrhea, and the above symptoms.

Food and General Safety

Cancer compromises the immune system and this is further impacted by treatments such as chemotherapy or use of steroids as anti-inflammatory agents for specific diseases.

Help reduce the risk of illness and infections by following safe food-handling practices such as:

- Avoid unpasteurized cheeses and honey, fresh—squeezed juices and ciders.
- Avoid the following foods when raw or uncooked: seafood, meat, eggs, alfalfa sprouts, bean sprouts, and cookie or cake dough (raw eggs).
- Never add raw eggs to smoothies due to the risk of salmonella, shigella, or E-coli contamination.
- Choose fruits and vegetables that do not have bruises, spots, dents or mold.
- Clean and disinfect knives, cutting boards, dish rags, towels, or other utensils used in food preparation. This can be done in the dish washer at high temperatures, or use a disinfectant.

- Do not keep leftovers in the refrigerator for more than two days. Reheat food until steaming or freeze right away if not consumed.
- When in doubt, THROW IT OUT!
- Wash your hands often as well as your food, or peel it; wear gloves when handling food.
- Avoid contact with ill persons, those with open sores, coughs, fevers, especially if they are helping you prepare food.
- Avoid lettuce and other fresh greens completely when your white cell count is low.
- Never eat under-cooked meat or poultry.

Other safety precautions:

- NO rectal thermometers to prevent trauma such as fissures in an already friable perianal skin.
- Do not clean cat litter boxes or bird cages.
- Don't garden without gloves, due to pathogens in soil.
- Wash your hands thoroughly and often. Keep your hands away from your face/mouth to prevent the spread of pathogens (germs, microbes).
- Wash your teeth well and use a soft toothbrush and dental floss. Bacteria in our teeth will get to all parts of your body via the circulatory system and may cause disease, especially of the heart. Studies have shown that bacteria from our teeth can cause myocardial infarctions (heart attacks).

Does Sugar Cause Cancer?

Sugar is a form of energy for the body. Our body needs glucose to provide energy for all cells. It is unclear how much sugar can be unhealthful. "The dose makes the poison," said Paracelsus. Some people believe that cancer cells thrive in a high sugar environment.

According to Dr. Lise Alschuler ND et al., cancer cells are studded with insulin receptors and will use insulin to stimulate growth of cancer cells. Therefore, if one has insulin resistance or is pre-diabetic, sugar should be avoided.

It is known that being overweight can lead to cancer. For example, high levels of estrogen in adipose (fat) tissue have been linked to many malignancies, especially breast cancer. Brown fat in the abdomen is also a risk factor for cancer, especially of the colon and prostate. This brown fat can also compress the kidneys and cause them to shut down.

According to Dr. Pamela Peeke, "Visceral fat, also known as belly fat, interferes with liver function by hampering the processing of cholesterol and insulin. It may also compromise the function of other tissues and systems." Studies have found links between belly fat and capillary inflammation. This can contribute to heart disease and insulin resistance, which is a precursor to diabetes as well as the cause of fatty liver disease. Fatty liver can damage an already compromised liver if NE cancer has metastasized to the liver. Fatty liver increases the risk of liver cancer. (Quian, et al., 2005)

When liver function studies are elevated, ask your physician if you have evidence of fatty liver disease, as a diet low in fat and certain medications may help in delaying progression of this condition.

Supplements

Many patients, newly diagnosed with cancer, may be tempted to start taking excessive amounts of supplements such as vitamins, minerals, and herbs. Unfortunately, most of these supplements are not regulated by the FDA so doses are uncertain. Many herbs and supplements interact with some medications and may actually be harmful. Do discuss this issue with a knowledgeable physician or a nutritionist. If you are able to eat a healthy diet with a wide variety of fruits and vegetables, and do not suffer from nausea, vomiting or diarrhea, you are getting all the nutrients you need from the food you eat, and therefore, you do not need supplements except as indicated by your medical provider.

However, most NET patients will benefit from taking selected dietary supplements such as pancrealipase, omega-3s, probiotics, polyphenols, antioxidants, and vitamin D_3, especially if D levels are subtheraputic. Supplements should come from a reputable source.

Eating a healthy, balanced diet is the key to optimum health. According to many experts in the field, nutritional deficiency is the single most important cause of all disease, including not only chronic illnesses, but infectious ones as well. Cells must be functioning well or disease occurs. Cells malfunction when they do not receive all the nutrients they need to perform their complex and life sustaining tasks.

"Let thy food be thy medicine and thy medicine be thy food."
—Hippocrates

We Are What We Eat

Every cell in our body is affected by what we eat or drink. Unfortunately, there is a vast difference between a wholesome and nutritious diet which most of us grew up with and today's fast foods. Industrial foods are heavily processed and full of chemicals. They are, consequently, a detriment to our bodies. We have become a nation addicted to fast foods containing large quantities of fat, salt, sugar, and chemicals which may stay in the intestine, long enough to enter our cells and start the process of cell mutation.

Whenever possible, unprocessed, organic foods are best. Avoid sugar or delete it from the diet and stop consumption of alcoholic beverages. If possible, avoid meats, dairy, processed, grilled, and high sodium containing foods.

Five servings of fruit and vegetables per day is the current recommendation. Each plate should have 2/3 vegetables, fruits, grains, beans or other legumes. One third or less should consist of meat, chicken or fish. If one is vegetarian, tofu or tempeh, grains, and nuts, may provide protein. Your plate should be as colorful as possible. Chewing each bite 20 to 30 times aids digestion. It is best to not drink water with meals to prevent dilution of stomach acid and enzymes, according to the Optimum Health Institute which also recommends we eat raw foods, which may be a problem if one is on a low fiber diet or has problems with gas and bloating due to short gut syndrome. One can reduce this problem by taking Bean-O before eating these gas formers and taking simethicone (Gas-X) before eating. Cruciferous vegetables like broccoli, cauliflower, cabbage, and Brussels sprouts are known cancer fighters, as well as many fruits such as blueberries, acai and gogi berries, apples and bananas.

Absorption of fat soluble vitamins such as A, D, E, and K, as well as other important vitamins and minerals becomes a challenge and can be reflected by changes in nails, skin, and hair, especially if we have post-surgical short gut syndrome.

Chewable AquADEKS° or Bariatric Advantage° brands of fat-soluble vitamins are recommended as they have been molecularly altered for better absorption. Vitamin B_{12} is also recommended for those on somatostatin analog therapy or who have had partial or total gastrectomies. B_{12} can be delivered by intramuscular injection or sublingually, although the sublingual form may not be adequate to meet one's needs. Levels of this vitamin should be evaluated frequently to ascertain that adequate replacement is achieved.

Fatigue

The majority of cancer patients experience fatigue. This is true of most of us with NETs. The fatigue is not one that is easily dispersed with a nap or a full night's sleep. The fatigue in NETs is one of extreme or excessive whole-body tiredness that is unrelated or out of proportion to exertion. It may be acute or chronic and impacts quality of life. It interferes with activities that bring pleasure or add value to our lives. Most people around us do not understand this fatigue. They may think we are malingering or trying to escape our activities of daily living. Fatigue also impacts our caregivers as they begin to take over what was normally our role in the family. It, therefore, can produce fatigue in them.

No one knows the cause of this profound fatigue in cancer patients unless an acute cause is identified: infection, fevers with or without sweats, anemia, loss of part of a lung. Insufficient nutrient intake, depression, or the tumors themselves may cause the body to function in an overactive or "hypermetabolic" state. Cancer cells compete for nutrients at the expense of normal cell growth and metabolism. The ensuing loss of weight, poor or no appetite and fatigue are the result.

Other contributors to fatigue include: chemotherapy, surgery, radiation, and PRRNT. Drugs used to control symptoms and side effects such as nausea, vomiting, diarrhea can also cause fatigue. Electrolyte imbalances due to unrelenting diarrhea can lead to fatigue. Pain, insomnia, and depression can aggravate fatigue in a vicious cycle.

As cancer cells die with certain therapies, certain substances are released that may contribute to fatigue.

Cytokines may play a role in fatigue. Cytokines are natural cell products or proteins, such as the interferons and interlukins, that are normally released by white blood cells (the cells in the body that fight infection), as well as lymphocytes and macrophages that respond to infection. These cytokines carry messages that regulate other functions of the immune and neuroendocrine systems. If high amounts accumulate, they become toxic and can lead to chronic fatigue.

Lack of adequate sleep during nighttime can lead to napping and in turn, the development of sleep disturbances, such as frequent awakenings. Early waking is a common symptom of depression. Anxiety also plays a role in insomnia due to increase in energy demands.

Treatment depends on the cause. Treating the under-lying cause may help; but sadly, it is not always easy to know what the exact cause is. All possible causes must be assessed thoroughly.

Transfusions, oxygen as a supplement, and medications such as Epogen˚ (medication which increases red blood cell production), and stimulants such as Ritalin˚ and Provigil˚ may be prescribed and monitored by your physician.

Other causes can be managed on an individual basis.

How to combat fatigue:

Keep a diary of which activities or situations make fatigue worse or better and pace yourself accordingly.

Plan rest and sleep periods in order to recover your energy before undertaking a task that you know will cause fatigue.

Select activities that bring you the most pleasure and do those first. Let other activities go or ask for help from others.

Make use of physical therapy and use aids such as canes, trapeze bars over your bed to lift yourself.

Ask the American Cancer Society or friends to drive you to appointments or accompany you to them. They can help conserve energy by opening doors, provide company and assist by listening to your discussion with your medical provider.

Begin to develop the art of delegating.

Exercise as tolerated so you do not lose muscle mass. Do not exercise unless you have the permission of your medical team.

Wait 24 hours after a treatment before exercising.

Do not exercise if you have a fever, low blood counts, or if your bones are involved with NETs.

Monitor your medications as they may be contributing to your fatigue.

Drink at least 8—10 glasses of water or other liquids a day to maintain hydration and eliminate waste products of treatments that may be the cause of your fatigue. It has been estimated that the major cause of fatigue in those with or without cancer is dehydration, especially if you drink coffee (a diuretic) or are on medications that cause you to lose fluids (diuretics).

Eat a balanced diet (see nutrition section).

Use distraction techniques so you do not focus on fatigue, disease or treatment. Read, watch movies, and talk with friends, or use support groups to discuss your symptoms openly and get ideas on how others cope with issues you are facing.

Set limits on visitors.

Get rid of negative people in your life.

Work toward eliminating the tiring habit of worry from your life.

Direct your own activities.

Rest often. Short rest periods are better than longer ones.

Go to sleep at a regular time each night and nap when necessary.

Do not berate yourself for being tired but do face the fact that you are fatigued and take the necessary actions to handle it. (Rosenberg, M.D., et al., 2012)

Major Organs of Digestion

To fully understand the digestive process, the organs of digestion are outlined as well as added recommendations for obtaining the most from our food intake.

Mouth and teeth are responsible for two major processes, noting that digestion begins in the mouth.

Mechanical shredding: Chew food until it is in liquid form to enhance digestion.

Saliva: The movement of food within the mouth mixes with saliva and starts the digestive process. Salivary glands are responsible for the secretion of a starch-splitting enzyme called ptyalin. Undigested starch can cause gas formation. If medications produce a dry mouth, there are supplements on the market that replace saliva, as well as sugar free gum and lozenges to keep the oral mucosa moist.

Eating slowly and deliberately allows for the beginnings of good digestion and extraction of all the nutrients available in food. During digestion, proteins are broken into amino acids; carbohydrates (starches) are broken into simple sugars, and fats into the smaller fatty acids and triglycerides.

Keep your teeth and gums healthy to promote proper breakdown of food, to prevent gingivitis and decrease the risk of diseases that may affect the heart via circulation. The teeth are also affected by NE cancers carcinoid. It is not uncommon to have chipping or loss of teeth due to malabsorption of vital nutrients such as vitamin D3 and calcium, although the aging process itself can cause this as can pain medications in the form of lollipops. These contain sugar and can have a detrimental effect on the teeth. It is, therefore, imperative to brush the teeth after using these agents or at least rinse the mouth well with water. Try not to fall asleep with these agents in the mouth.

Esophagus: Swallowing triggers peristalsis and with the help of gravity moves food toward the stomach.

Stomach: the widest part of the digestive tube. It is a muscular-walled, J-shaped sac in which food is stored, churned, and mixed with gastric juices secreted by its lining. This process begins moments after food enters the stomach through the gastroesophageal junction.

Gastric juices include digestive enzymes and hydrochloric acid, which break down food and kill potentially harmful microbes. The smooth muscle layers of the stomach wall contract to combine and squeeze the semi-liquid mix of food and gastric juices.

The stomach wall has four main layers. These layers contain gastric glands, acid producing parietal cells, and zymogenic and lipase-secreting cells necessary for digestion. The entero-endocrine cells secrete gastrin and other hormones.

Pancreas: the head of this gland nestles in a loop of the duodenum. Its main body lies behind the stomach, and its tapering tail sits above the left kidney, below the spleen. Each day the pancreas produces around 2 2/3 pints (1.5 liters) of digestive juice containing enzymes that break down lipids (fats), proteins, and carbohydrates. The fluid flows into the main and accessory pancreatic ducts which empty into the duodenum.

Specialized beta cells of the pancreas are responsible for the production of insulin. Insulin regulates carbohydrate and fat metabolism in the body. It causes cells in the liver, muscle, and fat tissues to take up glucose from the blood, storing it as glycogen inside these tissues.

Brain: the hypothalamus region of the brain is responsible for maintaining and regulating metabolism, body temperature, thirst, appetite, sexual behavior and blood pressure. It is also the center for nausea causation.

Liver: generates heat, thus acting like the body's furnace, helping to maintain core body temperature. It changes glucose into glycogen and stores it as fat. It also converts glycogen, fats, and proteins into glucose and then can change these back into glycogen, proteins and fats driven by an individual's state of health or disease. The liver also stores fat soluble vitamins: A, D, E, K, as well as water soluble B_{12}. This amazing organ is also responsible for manufacturing bile and the cascade of clotting factors.

Gallbladder: Concentrates and acts as a reservoir for bile made by the liver. Bile salts emulsify fats so they can be absorbed in the small intestine. Those on Sandostatin* may develop sludge and eventually, stones; therefore, the gall bladder is usually removed as a prophylactic measure during surgery for NETs. Medications such as Actagall* (ursodiol) are also used to prevent sludge from becoming stones.

Small Intestine: divided into three sections: the duodenum, jejunum and ileum and is approximately 20-22 feet in length. This is where most of our nutritive elements are absorbed.

The gastrointestinal tract, home to billions of beneficial bacteria, is also a prominent part of the immune system and its surface area is estimated to be that of a football field.

Colon: The large intestine is the final part of the digestive tract and comprises three main regions—cecum, colon, and rectum. The cecum is a short pouch that links the small intestine into the colon, which is about 5 feet (1.5m) long. The colon consists of the cecum, appendix, ileum, ileocecal valve, ascending, transverse, descending and, sigmoid colon. The rectum, internal anal sphincter, anal canal, and external anal sphincter make up the rest of the digestive tract.

The colon changes liquid digestive waste products from the small intestine into a more solid form that the body excretes as feces via the rectum and anus. The primary function of the colon is absorption of water and minerals, salts, and production of healthy flora necessary to synthesize B and K vitamins (OHI Institute, 2011), (Gray, 1944).

To enhance the digestive process, it is recommended that one eat fermented foods such as kimchee and sauerkraut regularly and drink sufficient pure water for adequate maintenance of digestive juices and mucous membranes as well as to replace fluids lost by diarrhea.

Probiotics are discussed elsewhere and help maintain the normal flora of the intestinal system and enhance immune function.

Dietary Recommendations for NETs

Eat a diet low in fat in order to reduce steatorrhea (greasy, foul smelling stools that float and may indicate malabsorption), which may result from short bowel syndrome. Somatostatin analog therapy may also cause a decrease in pancreatic function, making a low fat diet imperative. A fatty diet can contribute to gallstones, as can somatostatin analogs.

Engage in positive conversation during meal times or consider eating your meals in quiet contemplation with full attention to the experience of taking in life-giving nutrients. Consider the sacredness of eating to honor the body.

Reduce or eliminate alcohol consumption.

Enhance the immune system by adapting an anti-inflammatory diet. About 20% of people find that the nightshade family of vegetables like potatoes, eggplant, tomatoes, and peppers cause inflammation in the body which can lead to joint pain. (Alschuler, et al., 2011).

Include omega-3 fatty acids, probiotics, polyphenols such as curcumin from turmeric root or grain and antioxidants which are critical to digestive health and proper detoxification in one's diet.

Maintain proper levels of vitamin D_3 supplement in your regimen. Every cell in the body has receptors for vitamin D on their surface. Vitamin D_3 maintains our blood and bone levels of calcium and phosphorus, supports immune function, promotes cell maturation and regulates inflammation. A deficiency increases the risk of cancer and autoimmune disease. Vitamin D_3 is used in the production of neurotransmitters in the brain and deficiency is linked to depression as well. It is necessary for maintaining gut homeostasis and healthy gut bacteria. Since absorption of fat soluble Vitamin D_3 can be problematic for carcinoid patients, getting regular blood levels and supplementing with D_3 (not D_2) can be helpful. Taking Vitamin D_3 with the evening meal increases bioavailability. If there are problems with oral supplements, Vitamin D can be given intravenously or by other routes. The range for vitamin D, 25-HYDROXY is 20-79. Having blood levels drawn for this vitamin is important if taking supplements: both to avoid toxicity and to ensure the desired range is achieved. Many researchers have postulated that having a Vitamin D level above 60 is ideal to prevent cancer growth. (www.vitamincouncil. org, 2012).

Your physician may prescribe pancreatic digestive enzymes, such as Creon. These help breakdown fats, proteins, and carbohydrates in those with a deficiency of pancreatic secretion of these digestive enzymes. This process is possibly due to partial pancreatectomy, short gut syndrome, or rapid intestinal transit time, as found in carcinoid syndrome. Treatment with Somatostatin analogs also may suppress pancreatic function.

Consider magnesium for leg cramps. Your provider can measure levels. Do not supplement unless you have a low blood level. Plain tonic water may also be of benefit for cramps.

Additional Diet & Healing Recommendations for NETs

- Consume sufficient but not excessive calories, unless weight loss is an issue.
- Eat a colorful diet.
- Emphasize plant and marine sources of fats.
- Reduce or eliminate refined, processed, and packaged foods. If you can't pronounce it, don't eat it.
- Let moderation be your guide, according to Roman author, Cicero.
- Cancer likes excess fat! To avoid cancer recurrence, diet should focus on maintaining an ideal body weight/BMI (Body Mass Index).
- Pre-diabetes is a major health concern in the U.S., and is defined as a blood glucose level that is higher than normal but not high enough to meet the diagnostic criteria for diabetes. (Adler, M. M.D., 2013)
- Avoid alcohol as it has been linked to many cancers, heart disease and can trigger carcinoid syndrome as can caffeine.

- DO NOT TAKE supplements or herbs while on chemotherapy until you check with your doctor. Some supplements may interfere with the effectiveness of treatment!
- Do not heat foods in plastic containers in microwave ovens and if possible do not use microwave ovens.
- Do not drink fluids such as water if they have been warmed by the sun as the chemicals in plastic are known to leach into the fluids in the bottles.
- Do not drink out of plastic or aluminum containers. (Alschuler, L., ND, et al., 2011).
- Many persons with NE cancer are unable to tolerate tyramine containing foods, common in fermented and aged products, such as certain cheeses, and processed foods: also see the "5 E's."
- Limit avocados to half a cup. Limit canned figs, raisins, raspberries, red plums, fava or broad beans, Italian beans, Chinese pea pods, bean paste, tofu, miso and soy sauce.
- Avoid seasoning condiments that are tyramine containing and always check labels for these ingredients.
- According to the Nutrition Action Newsletter, the Ten Super Foods For Better Health are:

    1. Sweet potatoes—the best vegetable one can consume as they contain a lot of carotenoids, vitamin C, potassium, and fiber. After cooking and mashing, can add your favorite spices such as cinnamon, nutmeg, cloves, cumin, coriander, paprika, or chili (not recommended for those with carcinoid syndrome.
    2. Mangoes—approximately one cup supplies 100% of a day's Vitamin C, one-third vitamin A and a good amount of blood pressure lowering potassium, and 3 grams of fiber. This fruit is less likely to have pesticide residues.
    3. Unsweetened Greek yogurt—non-fat, plain. It is strained, so even the low fat versions are thick and creamy. The lost liquid means that the yogurt that is left has twice the protein of ordinary yogurt:

approximately 18 grams in 6 ounces. Adding cereals, vanilla, or your favorite fruits will enhance flavor.

4. Broccoli—high in vitamin C, carotenoids, vitamin K, and folic acid. Add a spritz of lemon juice or hemp seeds for taste and added nutrition.

5. Wild salmon—the omega-3 fats in this fatty fish can help reduce the risk of sudden-death heart attacks. Wild caught salmon has lower levels of PCB contaminants versus farmed.

6. Crispbreads—whole-grain rye crackers such as Kavli™, Ryvita™, Wasa™, are loaded with fiber and are usually fat free. Use honey and cinnamon, stevia, or organic agave for sweetness if necessary. Avoid high fiber diets if you've had a small bowel obstruction.

7. Garbanzo Beans—Rich in protein, fiber, iron, magnesium, potassium, and zinc. Garbanzos are more versatile than other beans: Use on salads, make hummus out of them, use in stews, soups, mix with brown rice, couscous, bulgur or other whole grains as tolerated by those with diarrhea or gas/bloating. It's recommended to use Beano™ before eating any beans or other gas formers. Sprout briefly before cooking.

8. Watermelon—two cups has one third of a day's vitamins A and C, potassium and lycopene for only 85 fat and salt free calories. They are less contaminated versus other fruits.

9. Butternut Squash—loaded with lots of vitamins A and C, as well as fiber. Cook well before consuming. Can make soup out of this wonderful vegetable.

10. Leafy Greens—eat as tolerated, especially if you have diarrhea. Kale, collards, spinach, turnip greens, mustard greens and Swiss chard. These are powerhouses of vitamins A, K, C, folate, potassium, magnesium, iron, lutein, and fiber. Serve with lemon juice but avoid red wine vinegar as it may lead to flushing. (Nutrition Action Healthletter, 2012)

One may have to experiment with eliminating foods in order to prevent debilitating diarrhea which is caused by serotonin release. Working with a nutritionist who is knowledgeable about neuroendocrine cancer can be extremely valuable. (Alschuler, Lise, ND, et al, 2011).

Survivor(n.):

1. *Literally, from Latin: one who lives through.*
2. *One who refuses to give up, give in, or quit trying.*
3. *One who triumphs over insurmountable challenges and becomes a better person because of them, e.g., those living with neuroendocrine cancers.*

Impact of Diarrhea

Diarrhea is a condition not unique to NETs. It is found in many other cancers and other disease states.

Over 80% or more of patients with NETs experience chronic secretory diarrhea during the course of our disease. In those who have carcinoid syndrome or short-gut syndrome due to removal of diseased bowel, diarrhea has the most impact on quality of life. It often renders the person homebound or ever on the search for bathroom facilities if away from home. In NETs, diarrhea is often accompanied by cramps, bloating, and explosive gas and stool. It can also be caused by side effects of treatments such as chemotherapy, radiation to the lower abdomen, food intolerances or infections, such as with clostridium difficile, often acquired during long hospital stays and/or treatment with antibiotics. Stress may also be a contributing factor.

The diarrhea of carcinoid syndrome mimics that of irritable bowel syndrome, leading to the most frequently misdiagnosed disease in NETs. Malabsorption can and does occur with protracted diarrhea. This state may lead to multiple problems with absorption of nutrients, vitamins and minerals. Malabsorption becomes yet one more problem that significantly impacts our lives.

Hormone mediators which cause diarrhea include serotonin, histamine, glucagon, prostaglandins, vasoactive intestinal polypeptide (VIP), gastrin, and calcitonin. (Anthony, L.B., 2004).

Some patients may experience steatorrhea (frothy, greasy stools that float), due to fat malabsorption. (See "organs of digestion"). It can occur in patients with pancreatic NETs such as somatostatinoma. It can worsen as the tumor advances or lessen if the tumor is resected or otherwise treated. Octreotide reduces diarrhea. Treatment with pancreatic enzymes is useful to increase absorption of fats, carbohydrates, and proteins.

Diarrhea can cause dehydration and electrolyte imbalance which can rapidly lead to a grave and even life-threatening situation.

Therefore, timely action is necessary to prevent complications. If one is unable to control diarrhea with conventional treatments, a home remedy of sugar and salt will help until medical help is sought. A good general formula is: 1 quart (liter) boiled water, 1 teaspoon (5 ml) salt, 1 teaspoon baking soda, 4 teaspoons sugar and flavor to taste. Check with your doctor to see if you can tolerate these particular ingredients. See your doctor as soon as is feasible for IV hydration and replacement of lost electrolytes/minerals and control of diarrhea. Further investigation may be necessary to rule out other causes.

There are simple actions that can be taken at the beginning of a diarrheal episode which may help reduce symptoms. Taking only liquids by mouth and avoiding solid food and milk may be helpful. Congee (rice porridge) is a semi-solid food that helps control diarrhea. It consists of white rice, boiled until soft, and taken an ounce at a time as tolerated. Nutmeg may be useful, as well as black raspberry powder with fresh turmeric and ground nutmeg added. Over the counter anti-diarrheals, such as Pepto-Bismol˙, Kaopectate˙, or Imodium˙ may also be of benefit. For explosive or persistent diarrhea, rescue with subcutaneous octreotide, and with a prescription and directions from your doctor, small doses of tincture of opium will stop diarrhea almost immediately, without any psychoactive or addictive effects. Diarrhea that stops when a proton pump inhibitor (PPI) is used is very suggestive of a gastrinoma. Somatostatin analogs inhibit pancreatic enzyme secretion and the absorption of fluid and nutrients by the intestine. NETs can produce diarrhea by different mechanisms, depending on what they secrete. (Vinik, et al., 2010)

For more information on the cause of diarrhea that is specific to you, discuss this issue with your healthcare team.

Caloric, electrolyte, and protein replacement is essential due to the loss of these nutrients during episodes of diarrhea. Supplemental vitamins and minerals such as calcium, magnesium, and iron can be taken once diarrhea is controlled.

THE GOAL WHEN HAVING DIARRHEA:
STAY HYDRATED!

Medium chain triglycerides (MCT), an oil that conserves lean body tissue, can be used as an alternative to conventional fat sources for easier and quicker absorption, and can be found in many health-food stores. In some people, these oils may cause diarrhea, so one is advised to start with small amounts and increase to tolerance. It is wise to take all supplements with a meal.

The use of black raspberry powder is an excellent way to control diarrhea and is reputed to have an anti-angiogenic effect on tumors. There are multiple sites and blogs that advise one on how to take this powder. (see Lucy Wiley's blog for instructions on it's use.)

Effective treatment depends on finding the cause of diarrhea. A good general approach is to keep a food and bowel movement diary and limit the diet to fluids for a few days to allow the bowel to rest.

Mild liquids can eventually be consumed: diluted fruit drinks (drink no more than 2 ounces at a time and wait at least 30 minutes before continuing to drink), common electrolyte replenishing drinks or electrolyte water, ginger ale, diluted peach or apricot nectar, water and weak tea may be tried initially. Hot and cold liquids or foods tend to increase intestinal muscle contractions and thus make diarrhea worse, therefore, these replacements should be warm or at room temperature. Carbonated drinks should be allowed to lose their carbonation before drinking, as they can cause abdominal distention and bloating which may lead to more diarrhea.

Frequent small meals will be easier on the digestive tract as well as low-residue nutritional supplements. Foods that aggravate diarrhea should be avoided: fatty, greasy and spicy foods, chocolate, coffee and all drinks containing caffeine. Other foods to consider avoiding: citrus fruits or juices, foods high in insoluble fiber or sugar, such as whole-grain breads/cereals or desserts. Avoid nuts, seeds, coconut, and legumes. Avoid fresh or dried fruit and prune juice. Avoid raw vegetables, popcorn, pretzels, potato chips, pastries, strong spices (except nutmeg). Avoid milk and milk products, though some can tolerate buttermilk and yogurt.

Potassium, a necessary electrolyte/mineral is also lost with diarrhea, as is sodium and magnesium. Potassium is necessary for heart and nervous system functioning and must be replaced. Foods high in potassium include bananas, apricots and peaches, potatoes (especially the skin if pureed), tomatoes, broccoli, halibut, asparagus, and, if tolerated: citrus juices, colas (allow to go flat), and low fat milk. Intravenous supplementation may be required, especially if the diarrhea is associated with vomiting. If there is no nausea and vomiting, the oral route (tablets or liquid) is preferred for supplementation. Some advocate the use of enemas for replacement, especially with wheat grass juice. If the ileocecal valve has been removed, colonics for cleansing are prohibited, but enemas are allowed.

After an acute episode of diarrhea, foods low in roughage/fiber and bulk should be gradually added. Steamed white rice or congee, cream of rice, banana flakes, applesauce, mashed potatoes without milk or butter, dry toast and crackers without salt are examples. Eat foods at room temperature.

Avoid alcohol, caffeinated drinks as in colas, coffee, and black tea, since these can worsen diarrhea and aggravate dehydration.

BRATT Diet

The BRATT diet has been around for years and is useful when diarrhea is a major problem.

- B—bananas, mashed to a fine consistency
- R—rice, congee or white
- A—applesauce
- T—weak tea initially as diarrhea lessens
- T—toast without butter or jam

Low in fiber and easily digested, these five foods have the ability to slow down intestinal activity and bind stool, thereby, stopping bouts of diarrhea. Depending on the cause of diarrhea, eating these gentle foods is a good place to start until the episodes subside. Other foods that are also low in fiber and helpful for stopping diarrhea include pasta, soda crackers and cooked cereal. Whole grain cereal is not advised, however.

Medications for Diarrhea

There are many over-the-counter and prescription medications available to control diarrhea. Work with you doctor or nutritionist to find what works best for you and reevaluate if not effective. You may need to try several agents before finding what is best for you. Some examples of anti-diarrheals include Lomotil*, Imodium*, Kaopectate*, paregoric (tincture of opium), cholestyramine (Questran˚). When single medicines fail, try Metamucil˚ plus Kaopectate˚ or alternate Lomotil˚ with Imodium˚ every other day. If Metamucil˚ is used, make sure you drink at least 1-2 glasses of water with it to prevent constipation. The aim is to add bulk to the stool, not form an immovable plug!

Many anti-diarrheals need a prescription from your doctor. These medications are dose dependent according to the prescriber. (Cancer Therapy Guide, Revised, 3rd edition)

Never ignore a gut feeling, but never believe that it's enough.
—Robert Heller

For this is the great error of our day that the physicians separate the soul from the body.

—Hippocrates (460-370 B.C.)

Complementary and Alternative Medicine

There is a broad range of complementary and alternative therapies for those with cancer or other life threating illnesses. The important distinction is the word "therapy," versus "treatment." Complementary and alternative medicine (CAM) addresses multiple side effects of cancer including pain, fatigue, nausea, and many other symptoms that are patient-specific. Always speak with your physician before availing yourself of CAM as some of these therapies may interfere with standards of treatment or even be harmful. Complementary and alternative medicine should never be used as a replacement for scientifically proven treatment options for cancer. There are many books written about personal success using CAM on an individual basis for symptom relief.

Some complementary and alternative treatments are listed below without endorsement by the author:

Acupuncture—A traditional Chinese medical approach employing the use of needles in certain points along the body's meridians used to relieve anxiety and pain, as well as to balance energy (chi) to promote healing. Traditional Chinese medicine can also include moxibustion, herbs, massage, exercise, and dietary therapy.

Diet and Nutrition—Many patients with cancer embrace a macrobiotic diet as a means to cure. The recent advents by Dr. Andrew Weil and Dr. Pritikin about the healing property of foods have lead many with cancer to take the route of nutrition as a healing agent. Many with cancer advocate a raw vegan diet or homeopathic supplements.

Nutrition is a viable and proven "treatment" of general health. The author recommends that before anyone embarks on a diet that claims to "cure" cancer, they speak to a specialist in this field.

Massage—Relaxation, pain relief, movement of lymphatic fluids and circulation. Touch is a powerful healing modality. Massaging areas over tumor sites should be avoided.

Medical Cannabis—Multiple states have restored the 5000-year medical use of cannabis, which was in the official United States Pharmacopoeia until 1942.

http://bit.ly/WDvWK9

However, cannabis remains as illegal as heroin (Schedule I—no medical use) under federal law, despite the fact that in all recorded history, there's no recorded instance of a fatal overdose. To add to the confusion, the U.S. Government itself, as represented by the Department of Health and Human Services, owns a 2003 patent on the medical benefits of cannabinoids:

http://1.usa.gov/14Mn2M9

Where state laws have been implemented, use of products derived from cannabis must be sanctioned by a medical doctor and does not exempt the patient from federal prosecution, which could result in lengthy prison sentences:

http://bit.ly/XwMIGo

Although medical cannabis research is in its infancy and is severely hampered by the legal climate in the United States, there is provocative evidence to support stimulating our body's own endocannabinoid system to aid in controlling, and possibly eliminating, cancer. Cannabis, or some of its over 400 known components such as cannabidiol (CBD), have also been used as an analgesic, to control nausea, reduce anxiety (including PTSD), treat anorexia, and to promote sleep.

Additional information can be found here:

www.medicalcannabis.com

http://www.cannabinoidsociety.org

http://www.ncbi.nlm.nih.gov/pubmed/16209908?dopt=Abstract

Anyone who hears that cannabis is a "cure" for cancer should know that such claims are, as of this writing, anecdotal in nature, not proven by double-blind, randomized, multi-centric clinical trials, and is therefore not accepted by the general medical community. While it's been said that the plural of "anecdote" is not "data", the sheer number of persons reporting benefit have provoked numerous ongoing research studies, both in the laboratory and clinically, throughout the international community. At the time of this writing, a PubMed search for scientific journal articles published in the last 20 years containing the word "cannabis" revealed 7,704 results. Add the word "cannabinoid," and the results increase to 15,899 articles.

Reiki—A Japanese technique for stress reduction and relaxation that also promotes healing. It is administered by "laying on hands" and is based on the idea that an unseen "life force energy" flows through us and is what causes us to be alive.

Reiki is usually administered by a "Reiki Master", one who has had extensive training in this form of healing.

Yoga—This ancient system stretches muscles that become tight due to a sedentary lifestyle or the disease process itself. It also helps the body to become limber and balances energy in the body, thus promoting relaxation. Injuries are common among those who fail to perform the asanas (positions) without mindful gentleness. Bikram yoga is practiced in a 110° F room and may cause flushing and other uncomfortable symptoms for those with carcinoid syndrome.

Tai Chi and Qigong—Qi, a Chinese character frequently translated as "life energy", literally means "air." Qigong practitioners consider good internal Qi flow as a necessary requirement and element of good health. Qigong is both meditative and incorporates a self-training set of movements which can lead to the control of one's Qi, and allow one to direct it to different parts of the body.

These exercises open up the meridians in the human body to allow the flow of energy to maintain health. Blockages are considered precipitous to the onset of disease.

Guided Imagery and Visualization—Guided imagery and visualization are techniques that, when practiced alone or with a teacher, can lead to peace and deep relaxation. Distancing oneself from inner body pain and "traveling" to a peaceful place may bring peace and relief of fear and anxiety. Some have used this technique to visualize disease states disappearing from one's body or disempowering the damaging consequences of a disease state.

Prayer—Regardless of one's religious beliefs, turning to a power greater than oneself and praying for healing has been shown to be a powerful tool for many. Having expectations and thinking positively can create a beneficial effect on the body, mind, and spirit. The old adage "you are what you think" allows one to appreciate the power of this belief system. Faith is perhaps the strongest belief we can use to give us hope which may lead to healing.

Meditation—Meditation fosters a state of consciousness in which the flow of concentration is uninterrupted. Benefits can include fostering the ability to release negative thoughts that interfere with sleep, appetite, and relationships with others. With meditation one can focus on healing, acceptance of one's state, and allow one to live in the present moment. Other benefits include quieting the mind of distracting chatter, enhancing the qualities of calmness, clarity, concentration and bliss. The term "carcinoid rage" is an example of uncontrolled feelings of anger which may occur without provocation and at inappropriate times. Meditation has shown to interrupt this state. (Chopra, 1993)

The reader is encouraged to find his or her own path to healing. Monthly journals such as CURE and HEAL are cited in the Resources section.

Emotional Health

"Lifestyle medicine" and behavioral modifications are increasingly important in managing our health, as we come to understand the integral nature of the body/mind.

Exercise as tolerated, especially if joint pain is experienced. Exercise should be nonviolent, such as walking or swimming, rather than heavy weight lifting or contact sports. Gentle yoga, T'ai chi ch'uan, and Qigong are highly recommended. A review of studies stretching back to 1981 concluded that regular exercise can improve mood in people with mild to moderate depression, even to the point of being an acceptable substitute for antidepressants. (Miller, Harvard Mental Health Letter, 2011).

Eliminate all negative emotions such as hate, envy, and jealousy. Especially avoid indulging in negative emotions or arguments during mealtimes.

Engage in forgiveness and gratitude.

> *Be kind whenever possible. It is always possible.*
> —Dalai Lama

Ask yourself, "Can I change this?" (Any situation one is worrying about). If the answer is "No," then worrying about it is unnecessary stress about stress! Useless. And if we *can* change the situation, we needn't worry: we need to take action! It's been said that worry is the opposite of prayer: it's praying for what we don't want to have happen.

> *Worry does not empty tomorrow of its sorrow; it empties today of its strength.*
> —Corrie Ten Boom

Worry is an utterly useless mental habit that can be eliminated by making a decision to change the habit, followed by repeatedly catching ourselves when we first go down that blind alley and practicing "erase and replace", i.e., gently shifting our focus onto what we *want* to have happen.

Make a pact with yourself about healthy coping. It is common to be worried and hyper-vigilant about our symptoms, but we have control over the mental habits that color our emotions. Life is about choice. Choose what serves *you* best!

Self-Advocacy

A diagnosis of cancer can spark many intensified feelings. It changes us physically, emotionally, and spiritually. It can instill emotions such as fear, anxiety, confusion, and vulnerability. One feels betrayed about living one's future, as we can feel our prospects suddenly taken from us and we find ourselves adrift in the fear of what will happen to us and our significant others. The stigma of cancer is ever present in our society, and pity for the person with cancer persists. This "soul pain" can be devastating and leaves us terrified of what is yet to come.

Cancer is a powerful life transition that asks us to question, explore, and transform our thought patterns and our lives. Taking time to explore these changes and feelings is as important to our health as rest, exercise, medication, and a healthy diet.

> *"Fear is a great accelerator of disease . . . Hope, faith, confidence and the will to live set an auspicious stage for recovery."*
>
> —Norman Cousins

Become Powerful!

A life threatening illness need not render us powerless. Instead, there exists a potential for life-changing experiences. One can transition into becoming a "peaceful warrior" and to take charge of our lives. Who else, besides oneself, has a greater dominion to take action on our behalf? Individually, only oneself can be depended upon daily to get the care needed in a timely manner and to speak honestly about our feelings and status. We resolve daily to bolster our spirits. Initially, it may seem that receiving a cancer diagnosis is insurmountable and overwhelming. Indeed, it is shocking to learn that our lives are now completely changed. The reality is that we have been given an opportunity to look within and heal what has been unaddressed for one's entire lifetime. The irony of cancer is that we can now choose to embrace our new reality versus feeling victimized and hopeless. There may not be a cure, but healing is always available.

Any cancer is a complex and manageable disease that needs one's full attention. My wish for you is that you gain hope, encouragement, and tools that will enable you to be your own best advocate.

HERE'S TO LIFE!

Get Organized

Enabling continuity of care becomes imperative as one meets with new and multiple doctors, given that many carcinoid patients will have several physicians during the protracted course of this cancer.

Record keeping is important in the continuum of care. Obtain copies of everything. This includes all laboratory work, imaging studies, pathology and surgeon's reports. A summary index sheet with dates of all tests from the date of diagnosis will be helpful to your multi-disciplinary team of providers, as well as to you.

Keep a journal of any changes in your symptoms or medications. This chronology will help you and your healthcare team track your cancer. Keep track of what makes symptoms worse and what relieves them. Have a designated place to record questions and concerns for your next appointment.

Self Education

Knowledge is Power!

The internet is a powerful source of information about our cancer. One can read articles from trusted sources related to NETs and watch videos by medical professionals discussing topics of interest. Learn the medical terminology so you can clearly communicate with physicians. They may take you more seriously if you are educated.

Be wary: everything you read on the internet is not accurate. Some articles may be journalistic or promotional advertising, and may be incomplete, outdated, or just plain wrong. There is a difference between anecdotal stories and medical evidence, as the saying shows: "The plural of 'anecdote' is not 'data'."

Question everything. When a doctor says, "This is inoperable", it may mean that either the doctor doesn't feel comfortable doing the procedure or he or she does not know anyone locally who would.

Such absolute statements should not be accepted blindly as truth. Often there are experienced surgeons who are familiar with your status and your needs that would perform a needed or recommended surgery. This is an example of where your record keeping will be invaluable. It also demonstrates how self-advocacy ties into the above.

Building Your Health-Care Team

Before engaging your physicians and other members of your integrative healthcare team, a powerful activity for you to consider: invest sufficient time to write your personal health narrative. This is like a novel, your story, about what has happened to you, with dates and places. Include all substances (medicines, herbs, supplements) you consume and results of tests and lab values. Look for insights: What have you discovered by reviewing your story? What is your recipe for self-healing as revealed by your story? Where would you like to change your story? What is *your* goal for *your* treatment? Write down whatever ending you want to choose.

Leave a copy of your whole narrative at each first encounter with members of your team, and bring updates to each subsequent visit.

If you are like many NET patients, you have already had contact with several doctors. You've already started your quest of what is best for you.

The most important activity in living with NETs should be consulting with an expert in the field. Neuroendocrine cancer is still considered a fairly rare disease by many, and treating it long-term requires access to the latest advances in the field. A NETs or carcinoid specialist may have seen hundreds of patients, usually in an academic "center of excellence" and has developed deep and broad experience in helping patients get answers for their needs. They have knowledge of the latest treatment modalities and educated expectations about challenges for your individual case. Several carcinoid websites have listings of NETs specialists by state.

After consulting with a NET specialist, take their suggestions for treatment to your oncologist. Have your primary oncologist become your ally.

You may have to interview multiple doctors before finding one that meets your needs. Take the time to research a potential doctor as to their training and the focus of their practice. Schedule a late-in-the-day appointment and let the scheduler know you are considering becoming a patient and would value some extra time. Ask relevant questions as to their training, experience, accessibility, how they handle emergencies, and who covers for them during vacation leaves. Be upfront with your own expectations and emphasize, perhaps most importantly, that you would like someone who is open to collaborating with a NET specialist. Ask if he or she is open to using a team approach.

Be open and candid with your questions. If your reading has left you puzzled, bring the article to your appointment so you can discuss it and have your questions answered. A good starting point in the initial visit is to ask if your doctor is willing to work with you in a collaborative manner.

Develop an open relationship with all providers. This includes receptionists and appointment schedulers. This will be of great benefit to you in the future. Accessibility to your medical team is one of the most important things you can develop. Ask for the best way to contact them. Use email and phone services but do not abuse them. There may come a time when you need easy access to your team of providers, and if you are labeled a "problem patient, the rapport you build with all won't work to your advantage.

If you are a member of a managed care organization, find out if they have an ombudsman, a patient advocate, or an advanced care nurse or case manager with whom you can work. Oftentimes, these "inside" people can navigate the system for you.

Be positive, proactive, and persistent in getting high-quality medical care. Be assertive but not aggressive. You deserve it. Your doctors work for you! Do not accept appointments that are offered weeks out when you have an urgent need. Avoid remaining in a doctor-patient relationship that has deteriorated to (or starts out as) being adversarial. Your doctor doesn't have to be your friend, but he or she needs to be your ally.

Preparing for a Physician Visit

One of the most important aspects of managing your cancer is regular visits to your doctor. Do your homework before you arrive at the clinic or office. It behooves you to have a written list of concerns, problems, changes in symptoms, and questions relevant to the time that has passed since your last encounter. You may want to update and review your narrative entries before your visit. Provide a copy for your physician to follow along. Take the opportunity at the beginning of your appointment to give the doctor time to review your records. Ask clear and concise questions from your list, starting with what concerns you most. Most doctors welcome your concerns, as it shows that you are in partnership with him or her and are involved in your own care. Consider changing physicians if your doctor consistently shows little interest in your queries and concerns. Being prepared circumvents confusion about your current status and precious time is not lost. You are entitled to know about treatment options for your particular disease, clinical trials, and most importantly, your prognosis. Do ask about the frequency of laboratory and imaging studies pertinent to your case. (Don't forget to ask for all copies for your records, once you have the results).

Studies have shown that 40 to 80% of medical information exchanged at doctor visits is immediately forgotten (McGuire, 1996). Of what *is* remembered, almost half is remembered incorrectly (Anderson, 1979). When one is anxious or on pain medications, retention is further impaired. You may want to have an advocate such as a partner or friend accompany you to your appointments. They can provide emotional support as well as record information you may have missed. You can also ask your doctor for permission to tape record the visit.

Avoid an organ recital: "my head hurts, I have a rash, my toenails have a fungal infection," et al. Pick, at a maximum, three issues you want your oncologist to address at your visit, as they have many patients to see.

Obtaining a second, third or more opinions is your right. Being a well-informed patient means all avenues of care for NETs are explored. This action can provide information unavailable to your primary provider.

Some Questions For Your Medical Provider

Questions for the provider are unique to the individual. Some of the more basic and which apply to everyone include:

• When should I call you?

- Ask about any new symptoms that have developed since you last saw your provider.
- Ask about current medications that no longer provide relief.
- When do I need to go to the Emergency Room?
- Can you refer me to a nutritionist knowledgeable about my disease?
- What are the side effects of the medications that you have prescribed?
- Are there any other ways I can prevent common symptoms?
- How much exercise do you recommend; what type and how often?
- Would you recommend alternative methods for coping with my symptoms? If so, what is your opinion about (name what treatment or treatments you may want to try). (Dollinger, et al., 1997).

Accepting Support to Promote Healing

This topic is probably one of the most challenging with a diagnosis of any type of cancer. Not everyone can or is willing to be open about their disease. The stigma of a cancer diagnosis may be one of the most potent limiting factors to the acceptance of help. However, there are many variables such as cultural background, religious beliefs, and feelings of vulnerability, as well as fear of being hurt by others when we open up our hearts. If one is open to sharing, the rewards of this interchange include peace of mind, a feeling of not being alone, and most importantly, the experience of group support is a powerful form of medicine. The benefit of healing of our heart space results from connecting with others.

You may choose to share or not. If you do, you may share only what is comfortable for you.

Talking to others gives them permission to ask questions of you, but you are in total control of what you are willing to disclose or not. It is alright to say, "I appreciate the caring behind your question, but I'm not comfortable sharing about that now."

If you are still working, plan for rest periods during your work day. This is especially important after treatments that may impact your functioning.

Many people in our lives will be inquisitive about our health and make inappropriate statements such as "but you look so good" or other comments that are hurtful. The reality is that in their ignorance, many well-meaning statements can be injurious to our spirit ("shin" in Chinese medicine). The truth is that they are asking because they care about us. Focusing on their love for us transforms these statements to a message of trust and acceptance. We begin to trust that we are loved.

A support group is another venue for sharing one's issues surrounding our cancer. There are several on-line groups listed in the Resource section of this book. Some are educational only and not intended for emotional support, while some offer both. Find one you're most comfortable with and share only what you're willing to. You can ask questions to learn, and, in turn, have the rewarding experience of assisting others out of your growing knowledge.

Safety First

Not only do you need to be your own self advocate, you also need to manage your cancer care. Be involved with all that will impact your disease. Being knowledgeable and managing events which may hinder your health may save your life. An example is someone who has an allergy to iodine. You must ask questions about the procedure and what medications are used before they are administered. An example is contrast media, which is given before CT scans. Barium used in someone who has had complications such as an ileus (bowel obstruction) mandates that you advise your medical team about this problem.

If you have other co-morbidities, such as diabetcs, be sure to inform all involved with your care, especially if you are going to receive contrast dye. If you have renal (kidney) impairment, you may not be able to withstand the nephrotoxic effects of contrast dye. This dye may cause a diabetic with renal involvement to go into overt kidney failure. If this status is known beforehand, you can be premedicated with an agent such as Mucomyst or other agents which protects the kidneys from contrast nephropathy.

Always carry information about the possibility of complications from invasive procedures which can lead to carcinoid crisis. Carry information on the proper treatment of carcinoid crisis.

Wear a medic-alert bracelet with information about your cancer, medications and allergies. You should also include information about who to call in the event of an emergency.

After Your Diagnosis

You find yourself in the middle of probably the worst crisis of your life. "Now what?" you may ask. This section will offer information that may help you move through this major life change.

After the initial shock and movement into acceptance, life goes on, albeit dramatically changed forever. You will embark on a journey that will give you the opportunity to grow spiritually and emotionally as you deal with the myriad issues of your particular form of NE cancer.

When you become aware of moving into a negative state, it's time to practice an exercise called "Erase and Replace." (OHI, 2011). This means that you transform negative thoughts into what you want to have happen. None of us can suppress the negative first thoughts or feelings that arise spontaneously. We *can* control subsequent thoughts and how to accept feelings so that they are not detrimental to us. In Alcoholic Anonymous, this is called doing away with "stinking thinking" or as the bumper sticker reads, "Don't believe everything you think". Guard your thoughts.

The one constant with NETs is that everyone is as unique as their disease. As you do your research, keep in mind that any stated statistics are derived from large numbers and do *not* apply to you as an individual.

Surround yourself with people who are optimistic. Disengage from negative ones. Read empowering books and anything that brings you pleasure. Make time for yourself. Journal writing is a powerful way to express emotions cathartically. Enjoy your favorite hobby or anything that brings you joy.

LIVE! Accept that this life-changing event is a gift, if one chooses to view cancer as a turning point. We have been given the opportunity to focus fully on what is truly important and that will enhance our lives, perhaps for the first time. Cancer is something we *have,* something we are *living* with, but not who we *are*. Not everyone is given the opportunity to fully embrace life and all that it offers. There are those who may be unable to accept the fact that life has now become an event that can bring us closer to ourselves and others. Accept that not everyone will feel as we do. Everyone is unique and entitled to their feelings.

We learn about compassion for self and others, as well as setting boundaries for ourselves. The potential power of a compassionate heart (deep appreciation of the emotions and experiences of ourselves and for others)—of trusting that we are loved—gifts us with power to transform the pain we encounter in this new phase of our development. What an extraordinary gift! (Epstein, L., 1999).

Transition to End of Life

A cancer diagnosis is a reminder of our mortality. All of us will die. We start the death process the moment we are born. Some of us will meet our demise earlier than others, but all living things culminate in the death process.

For most people with NETs or any cancer, a cure will not be possible. Although this cancer is slow-growing, if metastasis has occurred, is poorly differentiated, or if complications arise, we and our loved ones need to prepare for the inevitable. We may live a long time with proper management of our individual cancer or die from complications related to NETs. Some will succumb to causes not related to this cancer.

Our culture in the U.S. is not noted for its acceptance of the death process. We are in fact, afraid of death, distracting ourselves in our denial of the inevitable. Conversely, many of us have come to see that to die is as natural as living.

Family and friends experience a range of emotions when facing the impending death of a loved one. They too, share the shock and disbelief, as well as the feelings of anger and the overwhelming sense of helplessness to change the course of events. In some cases, there may be a sense of relief that the suffering and struggle is nearly over. Some may feel guilty for having these thoughts.

For some, the time before death comes can be one of strengthening relationships and creating lasting memories. This time offers an opportunity to share, in a deep and profound way, what their lives together have meant. Not everyone will be able to discuss these topics easily and may need assistance in doing so. Palliative care volunteers may be called upon for assistance as well as preparing for hospice. It is important to remember to focus on life and living until death comes. One needs to live fully until that time.

It is prudent to prepare in advance for this inevitability. This is also a loving thing to do for our families. It can be carried out with the assistance of a facilitator such as a therapist, social worker, a skilled hospice worker, or palliative care physician.

"Death is not a disease and dying is not a medical condition."
—Sherwin B. Nuland, MD

Hospice

Hospice is a philosophy of care that originated with Dr. Cicely Saunders in England during the 1950s. Her work focused on palliative care. This care is directed towards preserving quality of life and should begin from the time of diagnosis to the end of life.

The purpose of this care focuses on living with cancer while dying. It places the emphasis on physical, emotional, spiritual, and social needs. The physical often takes precedence, as it addresses pain and other symptoms that rob a person of quality of life. Family and friends are an integral part of the hospice team. Care is provided in hospitals, nursing homes, hospice centers, or the patient's home. The care is provided under the guidance of a physician medical director and a cadre of visiting nurses and home health aides as well as volunteers.

Hospice becomes part of a patient's final days with the patient's and family's permission. A referral to hospice services is usually made when a person has been told, that based on their symptoms, they have six or less months to live. There are times when a patient's condition stabilizes and they are able to leave hospice care and return to a pre-hospice level of functioning.

Under hospice care, usually no further treatments aimed at arresting disease progression are given except for palliative care. This care varies, as some states now see and allow blood transfusion or IV fluids as palliation. In many instances the primary care physician or oncologist may continue to visit. Conversely, care may be turned over to the medical director of the hospice facility. It may also be under the auspice of the hospice agency directing care in the home.

Caring Bridge (https://www.caringbridge.org) is offered on the internet to help families disseminate information about the status of a loved one who is too ill to answer questions about his or her condition.

Advanced Care Planning

Transition to end-of-life care is imperative, as it relieves the burden from loved ones and expressly implements the dying patient's wishes. While a will and/or living trust addresses estate issues, including finances and the distribution of one's assets, a durable power of attorney and an advance directive names one or more trusted individuals to carry out one's wishes with regard to care.

An "advance directive" is the document of choice and focuses more precisely on end-of-life issues. These issues need to be addressed in advance by discussing them with family members, a social worker, or medical professional and completing the document. An advance directive specifies one's decisions regarding final care. (See the Resources section to download your state's form or obtain one from your physician or medical facility).

Usually distinct but sometimes a subset of an advance medical directive is a do-not-resuscitate (DNR) order. This document is a patient's instruction to family and healthcare providers and addresses whether or not to attempt cardiopulmonary resuscitation (CPR) and other advanced life support measures in case of cardiac or respiratory arrest. Unlike the advance directive, a DNR must be signed by a physician in most states.

It should be stressed that, in the United States, an advance directive or living will is not sufficient to ensure a patient is treated under the DNR protocol, even if it is his wish, as neither an advance directive nor a living will is a legally binding document. It is also the case that the wishes expressed in an advance directive or living will are not binding. (http://en.wikipedia.org/wiki/Do_Not_Resuscitate).

A copy of these documents should be provided to your physician(s). It should be readily accessible for emergency technicians in the case of an event at home or while traveling. Many people place them on the refrigerator door and carry a small copy in their wallet. Those whom you have appointed as health care agents should have a copy as well.

An advance directive empowers the patient to maintain control in a dignified manner. Prior planning and self-advocacy bring relief to what inevitably will be a very trying time for everyone. This discussion should include loved ones or a trusted individual who will confidently execute the end of life care decisions. *Five Ways* is an easy, fill-in-the-blank document that allows one to specify end-of-life wishes. It can serve as a complete guide to declare both one's wishes and also appoints a Health Care Agent. Five Wishes can be obtained from Aging with Dignity at www.agingwithdignity.org or by calling 888-5-WISHES.

When to Call in Hospice

Hospice care is still the only answer at the end of life, when patients want to stay at home surrounded by the people they love and the things they cherish. However, it is important that hospice care is initiated while there is still time for the Hospice team to get to know the unique needs and wishes of the individuals and their families.

The dying process is the most intimate time, other than birth, that we all go through. The majority of us do not want strangers by our bedside unless absolutely necessary. When hospice is called in too late, it can feel very intrusive, and more like an Intensive Care Unit, where the role of the nurse is that of administering medication and following protocols, instead of being a trusted member of the family and community, who no longer needs to ask questions. No one knows when their time to die will come, and I feel that if an individual has made the decision to no longer go back to the hospital for treatment, then Hospice is a choice. You may believe that you have more than six months to live. However, Hospice can always be put on hold, if you get better, and restarted if your condition should change and you begin the transition phase into the dying process.

—Hanne Jensen-Male, Hospice and Palliative Care RN, and Certified Case Manager

In Switzerland I was educated in line with the basic premise: work, work, work. You are only a valuable human being if you work. This is utterly wrong. Half working, half dancing—that is the right mixture. I myself have danced and played too little.
—Elizabeth Kübler-Ross

The Steps Slowed

There she lay against the white pillow, so pale, so pale
Withered hands, wrinkled, so frail, so frail
Tubes emanating, jumbled from every orifice she had
Faded blue-grey eyes seemed flat, unfocused, scared?
Seemed to see behind me, through me, in a straight line
As if aware of the "Do not resuscitate" sign
That simple card that said so little, so much
Our society's final banishing touch

Day by day she weakened even more
I noted my reluctance to enter her door
Her feeding tube removed, I tried not to imagine
How her morphine smothered life was flagging
The normal banter of medical euphemy
Seemed stilted, uncomfortable, almost blasphemous
Even the seasoned attending's body system's checklist
Appeared perfunctory, the drone of a blind man's cane in a mist

Her family knew her time was close
They came in the elevator every day, those whom she loved
most
A sense of forced normalcy permeated the atmosphere in
the room
Tight, nervous laughter did little to dispel the gloom
If ever I was there when they came I felt shunned and outcast
They knew that the limits of medical knowledge had passed
I felt trapped, helpless and viewed like a hindrance and a
reminder
That ours were the tubes that uselessly coursed inside her

Unbelievably the days drew on, she stubbornly refused to
let go . . . till one night
After faithfully churning for eighty-four years her heart
went out like a light
I was the first doctor on the scene, alerted by the nurse
Close behind me a senior resident, who knew this was my
first . . .
Medical training at the forefront, all emotion was banned
A lesson in "how to certify death" summarily began
It helped somewhat that I was doing something seemingly
productive at last
The body shell was starkly robotic, the face just a mask

As the nurses fixed up the bed for viewing she would be ready
I learned how to fill out the papers, my training made my
hand steady
I headed outside the room, then heard the elevator bell
Knowing what it signified, it roared in my head like a
death knell
Saw the familiar family faces rushing out, their hope
flickered, then was dispelled
For so many weeks, this moment had been dreaded, with
all emotion withheld
Despite the certainty of the outcome the heart clings to the
comfort of the denial track
But seeing their faces crumple, was the straw that finally
broke my back

In those moments I was no longer Doctor White Coat, rejected
Death had shattered the shields which both parties had
erected
Intense emotion bursts its holding dam, as their steps
slowed hesitantly
This could have been my mother, my child, my partner,
even me
I sobbed with them as I grieved that wonderful feisty
spirit's passing and her grace

So much healing can be done with non-verbal communication taking place
And after our relationship, which weeks of malignant carcinoma had begun
I will never forget that final moment when every prejudice was lifted and we were all (including her) One.

—Lally Pia, MD August 22, 2011

Internet Resources

ACOR www.ACOR.org Association of Cancer Online Resources A forum for threaded discussions related to carcinoid cancer.

Advance Medical Directive: download your state's form http://www.caringinfo.org/i4a/pages/index.cfm?pageid=3289

American Cancer Society www.cancer.org

American Institute for Cancer Research www.aicr.org The New American Plate and Nutrition Information Center

Asia Pacific CNETs www.cnets.org Carcinoid Foundation from Singapore. Features patient information and videos by physicians

Australia—www.carcinoid.com/au Carcinoid Cancer Resources for Australians

Australia: Unicorn Foundation www.unicornfoundation.org.au The Unicorn Foundation is the only Australian not-for-profit medical charity focused on neuroendocrine tumors (NET).

Board and Web Site NET's www.netpatientfoundation.com Europe based discussion board. Discusses treatments available in Europe.

Breakaway from Cancer www.breakingawayfromcancer.com Resources on preventing, fighting, and surviving cancer

Cancer Adventures www.canceradventures.org Website focuses on helping survivors meet their needs in terms of nutrition, inspiration, resources for establishing a thriving survivorship program

CancerCare, Inc www.cancercare.org 800-813-HOPE CancerCare is a national nonprofit organization that provides free professional support services to anyone affected by cancer.

American Society of Clinical Oncology (ASCO) www.cancer.net ASCO provides oncologist-approved information about cancer. The web site can be viewed in English or Spanish

CancerCare www.cancercare.org Includes an especially good section on care giving

Cancervive www.cancervive.org/education.html See the caregiver section

Carcinoid Cancer Awarenesss Network www.carcinoidawareness. org Information and support to NET patients and caregivers, ho sts national conferences and presents them via online webinars for viewing

Carcinoid Cancer Foundation www.carcinoid.org Information about these diseases, including information about NET/carcinoid focused doctors around the globe, nutritional considerations, listing of community support groups, treatment, clinical trials and a wide variety of resources

Caring for Carcinoid Foundation www.caringforcarcinoid.org Dedicated to funding and discovering cures for NETs, resources, physician database, research, announcements of latest advancements and research

Clinical Trials www.clinicaltrials.gov US Government web site detailing clinical trials

CNETs Canada (Carcinoid Neuroendocrine Tumor Society) www. cnetscanada.org

Consensus Guidelines for the Diagnosis of NETs from NANETs nanets.net/pdfs/pancreas/03.pdf

ENETs www.neuroendocrine.net European NET focused site. In English. Education, trials, publishes treatment guidelines, annual conferences. Managed by European Carcinoid NET MDs

Germany www.net-shg.de In German. The federal self-help organization of Germany

Germany-Network Neuroendocrine tumors www.glandula-net-online. de In German, information, support, conferences for patients and caregivers

InterScience Institute www.interscienceinstitute.com A diagnostic laboratory focusing on NeuroEndocrine Tumors. They have published *Neuroendocrine Tumors: A Comprehensive Guide to Diagnosis and Management* which is available via a downloadable pdf file or printed by request

Live Strong www.livestrong.org Lance Armstrong's Foundation helps people with cancer and their loved ones through advocacy, education, public health, and research

Lucy's Blog www.lucysnoidblog.blogspot.com Lucy, a carcinoid patient posts information and insight relevant for NE cancer patients

Medline www.nlm.nih.gov/medlineplus/ Comprehensive medical dictionary run by the National Institute of Health

Memorial Sloan-Kettering Cancer Center www.mskcc.org/cancer-care Help for Caregivers, Families & Friends

NANETs—North American Neuroendocrine Tumor Society—www. nanets.net US NET/carcinoid medical society, whose purpose is to improve neuroendocrine tumor (NET) disease management through increased research & educational opportunities. Coordinated by US carcinoid physicians

National Cancer Association www.nccn.org Devoted to patients, caregivers, and family, the only patient-oriented cancer website based on the NCCN Guidelines™ which set the standard of care for clinicians around the globe.

National Cancer Institute Caregiver Information: http://cancer.gov/cancertopics/coping/when-someone-you-love-is-treated

National Coalition for Cancer Survivorship—www.canceradvocacy.org.info and resources on cancer support, advocacy, and quality of life issues

NET ALLIANCE www.thenetalliance.com Information, support, and insights for people affected by neuroendocrine tumors A Novartis Pharmaceutical sponsored site

NET Patient Foundation www.netpatientfoundation.com Downloadable booklets, information, resources, physician database for USA & UK/Europe, links. Sponsored by pharmaceutical companies

Patient Advocate Foundation www.patientadvocate.org Education, legal counseling, and referrals to survivors concerning managed care, insurance, financial issues, job discrimination, and debt crisis issues

Society for Integrative Oncology www.integrativeonc.org—Advancing evidence-based, comprehensive, integrative healthcare to improve the lives of people affected by cancer

Strength for Caring www.strengthforcaring.com (site owned by Johnson & Johnson)

Sunny Susan Anderson www.carcinoidinfo.info The first personal website by a carcinoid patient, details her journey through carcinoid with educational resources available

Sweden—Carpa www.carpapatient.se—In Swedish. An educational association in Sweden

The Cancer Info Web Site www.cancerlinksusa.com—Includes links to financial help organizations, recommendations for first steps after diagnosis, medical oncology terms dictionary

The Insurance Warrior www.theinsurancewarrior.com—Laurie Todd is a health insurance strategist. She writes insurance appeals. Her site offers tips on researching, writing, and delivering a winning appeal, offers appeal-writing services. She has written two books on the subject.

The Wellness Community www.thewellnesscommunity.org

U.S. Department of Agriculture www.fnic.nal.usda.gov National Agriculture Library, Food

U.S. Food and Drug Administration www.fda.gov

Well Spouse Association www.wellspouse.org

Yahoo Groups www.groups.yahoo.com/group/CARCINOID-ACOR A threaded discussion group for carcinoid education. Registration required. Monitored by Dr. Woltering at LSU-Kenner

The National Organization for Rare Disorders, an alliance of health organizations which maintains a database with information about a multitude of rare diseases and related health advocacy and information groups at www.rarediseases.org or call 800-999-6673

The National Institutes of Health's Office of Rare Disease Research offers an online gateway to a host of information links related to rare diseases, including rare cancers, at www.rarediseases.info.nih.gov, or call 888-205-2311

More resources:

www.curetoday.com/toolbox

HEAL magazine—free to those with cancer.

Carcinoid Coffee Cafe support group via Facebook

Zebra Zone support group via Facebook

Carcinoid Awareness support group via Facebook www. newlifestyles.com www.ncl.nih.gov/cancertopics/coping/ familyfriends http://thesecondopinion.org/

The mission of thesecondopinion.org is to provide free multidisciplinary second opinions and related services to adults in California diagnosed with cancer.

How to donate to NET Awareness Programs

Donations to the Carcinoid Cancer Foundation can be made by check or credit card. Please make checks payable to the foundation and mail to The Carcinoid Cancer Foundation, 333 Mamaroneck Avenue #492, White Plains, NY, 10605 or visit the foundation's website, www.carcinoid.org to make donations online by credit card.

Consider these fine organizations who contribute so much to our cause:

www.carcinoidawareness.org
www.caringforcarcinoid.org

Thank you for your donation on behalf of all
NET and Carcinoid patients worldwide.

Survivor and Caregiver Stories

Why stories?

Through time, stories have taught us many things through context and example. By visiting our doctors, rare windows sometimes open and shine briefly upon the naked human spirit. Here, we as outsiders can have a glimpse into those intimate moments shared between doctor and patient, as well as family members.

As a musician effortlessly moves among notes and phrases to produce a rich and exciting sound, so do stories that come from the heart. These are not improvisations but memories instilled and written on the heart. Stories about what works and what doesn't work remind us of what is important and keep us centered and grounded. These stories are as close to the truth as words and remembrance allow. Stories are an opportunity to trace the human spirit through their journey. I am fortunate and thankful to our contributors for allowing me to share these intimate accounts.

These contributions are left largely intact as provided and only briefly edited. I chose to honor each individual and leave their "voice" intact as written.

Maria Gonzalez

Maria's Wild Ride

A cancer diagnosis catapults us down a slippery, surreal rabbit hole into a world where we are stripped naked, powerless and fear-filled. I had been diagnosed with breast cancer in 1989 and underwent a lumpectomy, followed by radiation. I said "no" to tamoxifen as the odds that it would be of benefit were 2%. I was diagnosed with tubular, infiltrating ductal carcinoma, and if one "wants" cancer of the breast this is the one to have: slow growing, and mine was the size of a tiny pea.

Five years after my ordeal with breast cancer with the daily visits for six weeks to the radiology department at UCSF—watching the bald heads, the blank looks in vacant eyes, the young ones wheeled into the basement where radiology was located, the IV poles—(drip-drip . . .), the dressings covering oozing, never healing lesions of cancer, the drug muffled pain. I sensed their fear, mixed with my own; the Grim Reaper waiting in the dark shadows of the windowless rooms in radiology. Little did I know I was to encounter cancer yet again.

I had gone dutifully for my treatments, to receive the same poison that caused deformities in Nagasaki and Hiroshima, the same rays from the sun that can cause skin cancer, but also give us our Vitamin D and cause beauty to grow all around us. On my treatment days, I would run the five miles to UCSF from home and back. I planted a garden and pulled weeds with a ferocity. I imagined I was pulling out cancer by the roots. I walked in Golden Gate Park and talked to God to let me live a few more years to do His work.

Listen to your favorite music, I was advised! Music! What music? My heart's quick beating, the river of sweat running down my back, the voices in my head telling me I was a goner? Strawberry Fields Forever this was not . . . more like Jimi Hendricks, The Wind Cries Mary (Maria). I surrounded myself with an imaginary leaden shield to prevent collateral damage to other organs in my body. I saw the blinking light of the "radiation monster" as the eye of God, healing me.

I thought I was done with cancer, only to learn that after years of fatigue, generalized bone pain which came out of the blue and which I blamed on my marathon running and cardio-kick-boxing as the cause, once again, the vulture of cancer came calling. I liken it to crows in broad daylight, fearless as they eat the young seedlings I planted in my garden. My bone scan was negative, so why all these strange symptoms? Why did the word "liver" keep popping up in my mind? I felt I was once again dodging bullets from a predator—running through a jungle in fatigues, well camouflaged. I obviously was not well camouflaged. Cancer had found me again.

I started having early satiety, weight loss, my gastrointestinal tract started grumbling as though to say, "Hey, help me, something is very wrong". "Pay attention to me!" I looked the other way, but my inner self knew there was another invader in my body.

One night, as I ran with my friend Marjie and my partner Bill, I was stricken with a pain in my left flank, so strong it brought me to the ground. They kept talking, thinking I was stretching as I knelt on the ground. Eventually, I managed to get their attention and was brought home to a hot bath, a 5 mg. tablet of Valium˙ and half a beer to relax my muscles. I began reeling from the possible causes for my signs and symptoms—a muscle strain/sprain, a urinary tract infection, a renal stone lodged in my ureter? Eventually I fell asleep, and the next day asked a radiology friend what the best modality was to diagnosis a kidney stone. He quickly picked up on the fact that the patient I was talking about was me and he said, "Jump on the helical scanner and let's have a look." With trepidation I did, and as we reviewed the images, I saw multiple lesions in my liver. David did not seem concerned and I insisted we review them again. That is when he remembered my past history of breast cancer and before I knew it, I was in the very emergency room where I worked on weekends. The nurses were amazing, maintaining my privacy in a private room as I was readied for a CT with contrast. My colleagues in the clinics where I worked came down to the ER to be with me as I freaked out. Not again, not mets. None of my fellow colleagues were impressed with the results of these liver lesions. All they could tell me was, "They are not mets from your breast cancer and you have no evidence of any other lesions anywhere." What then? My mind randomly raced. It was like a fluorescent bulb going on and off, sometimes flickering in between.

What ensued was a chase of my radiology friends in various institutions. None could tell me what those strange and unwanted visitors to my liver were. Dr. E. knew that I had not had any tests other than my CT scan. The octreotide scan would come later.

I went to my regular oncologist, head of the Oncology Department of a large hospital in a major city, but he laughed at my suggestion that there was something strange going on in my body. Even with my diagnosis of breast cancer, he had never scanned my chest, abdomen or pelvis, all for the sake of saving the expense and getting his kudos from his fellow MD's and corporate managers. He concluded I had irritable bowel syndrome, and, over the next year, variously called me neurotic, a closet alcoholic, a somatizer, menopausal, ad nauseum! I must be merely stressed out and imagining things. "Hysteria" he called it! How dare this pompous man talk down to me! I felt a surge of anger rush through me and I wanted to hit him. How dare he not listen to his patient and investigate my symptoms? At least he did not offer me a vibrator as they would prescribe in olden times.

I have a wonderful friend and colleague who is an endocrinologist. He suggested I might have carcinoid, as by this time I was flushing and looking like a cooked lobster. Any activity set off the flushing: dancing, exercise, stress, foods, coffee, and emotions. My friend Marty suggested I tell my doctor to run a 5-HIAA and a CgA. Reluctantly, just to shut me up, my then oncologist ran the tests and both were positive. Three liver biopsies later, I had the diagnosis of adenocarcinoma of the liver with features of neuroendocrine cancer. Our hospital pathologist verified the diagnosis and I saw the sadness in her eyes, the compassion. My fear intensified.

With this new diagnosis of carcinoid, I knew only what we had done for L., the only carcinoid patient ever seen by the oncologist with whom I worked. Little did I know what lay ahead: a protracted cancer, lurking in the dark, Close To The bone, as Dr. Jean Shiboda-Bolen describes in her book by the same title, in my marrow, waiting to take advantage of my frail body and mind if I let it.

This second encounter with cancer was with a relatively rare and misunderstood form. Being in nursing and then in medicine, I had seen only one case of carcinoid in 20 years of practice. My colleagues admitted they had heard of it, but only briefly and had never seen a case, until L. came to see Dr. E. in oncology clinic. I recall feeling sorry for her and moving on, wiping my brow that I did not have her kind of cancer. L's symptoms were unrelenting diarrhea, weight loss and fatigue. I saw this beautiful woman drop her weight from 145 pounds to a mere 95. She was admitted to our long term care ward after a bowel resection and maintained on Sandostatin˚. This drug did wonders for her symptoms, but she was left with short gut syndrome, and she eventually had to be fed via a tube directly into her body (total parenteral nutrition). She died of line sepsis (infection) from the IV catheter for her feedings. Before her death she copied information on carcinoid for us, scarce as it was, but I did NOT read it. I gave it a cursory glance. It was her issue, not mine, and Dr. E. was handling her treatment, as was our endocrinologist. Little did I know what lay in store for me.

The word "cancer", with its stigma of death, propelled well-meaning friends and relatives who do not understand the trauma they inflict, to tell me about some relative or friend who died a horrible death due to cancer, as they made the sign of the cross ("May it not be me", they uttered under their breath). They unknowingly cut into my core, deepening the wound already draining my life force.

I went to "why me?" What did I do now to deserve this? I blamed myself for the stressful life I lived. The whirlwind of medicine is a demanding mistress and I danced the dance: eating my lunch in 10 minutes, gobbling down a lean cuisine in 15 minutes if I were lucky, the entire time signing my charts on the computer, answering patients calls, re-filling prescriptions, moonlighting in the emergency room or the racetrack on weekends, twelve hour shifts with barely time to eat standing up, never mind using the toilet. At the end of the day, I ran out of the hospital clinics and went straight to the gym to cardio-kick box or run around a lake in San Francisco. I would come home beat, in horrific total body pain, to a hot shower, which eased the pain. My partner would have dinner or I would throw something together and we would eat around 9 pm.. Time to check e-mails, answer personal phone calls, read mindless novels in bed and lucky me if I turned the lights off at midnight, only to get out of bed by 6 the next morning, ready to commute 26 miles to work and join the dance again! My partner's concern went unheeded. Stress, what stress?

Eventually, despite my oncologist's assurances of it being "indolent," I got that this was one cancer I could not ignore and began a self-study in the treatment of carcinoid. I read books, joined two support groups and called people to see how and what they had done to deal with this strange cancer. My nurse friend Donna, Bill and I attended a pharmaceutical dinner where I met Dr. Rodney Pommier. The topic was carcinoid cancer, and of all the physicians, oncologists and surgeons, who had RSVP'd in the San Francisco Bay Area, we three were the only ones who showed up. From Dr. Pommier, and also a convention on carcinoid cancer held in Portland, Oregon, I learned that surgery might help delay the progression of the disease by finding and removing the primary tumor in my midgut. I learned that this cancer is usually detected only at an advanced stage where treatment is rarely curative. It is equally quiet on another front—historically, there have been few headlines extolling breakthroughs in the treatment of this neuroendocrine cancer. My oncologist, just before I fired him, said there was no reason to have surgery, that it was not supported by double-blind prospective studies, and that Dr. Pommier's published data was retrospective only and therefore of no real use.

In 2008, I traveled to Portland, Oregon to undergo debilitating surgery (removal of 9 tumors in my liver, leaving two behind due to blood vessel encasement, 18" of small intestine plus my gall bladder). It was a horrendous surgery, complicated by a liver abscess on my return to San Francisco, as well as an infected incision, along with a raging C. difficile infectious diarrhea, a complication from the antibiotics during my recuperation in the local hospital.

Bill is a nurse and he patiently nursed me back to health, emptying the bile drainage, changing my dressings twice a day, packing and washing my two infected, now open wounds (4 inches and 10 inches long) until I grew stronger and returned to work. I was told to take 6-8 weeks off. I went back after four weeks, ever loyal and seeking approval, convinced that only I could take care of my patients! Ego involvement? You bet!

I was working to smother the adrenal-squeezing fear which enveloped my every waking moment. If I took care of others, I did not have to feel my feelings, especially "cancer", fear of the unknown, of death. I was filled with anxiety and depression, knowing full well that these feelings were damaging my immune system even more. But I was taught to not show my feelings, to pretend all was well when it was not—when my father came home drunk and out of his mind, with my mother, so focused on his drinking and trying to change him. I learned early on to be the parental child, to take care of all except myself. No wonder I went into the helping profession: validation from outside vs. inside.

The death of my beloved brother ten days after he came home from Vietnam: the spark of who he was, his beautiful life gone in the blink of an eye, threw me into a life of not caring whether I lived or died. I even contemplated suicide! My younger brother drank himself to death at age 35, and my family fell deeper into the abyss of nowhere land, unable to process the myriad of feelings we all suffered in silence.

My life became a series of jobs and parties, multiple lovers, drugs and alcohol, angry outbursts at friends and the world, swallowing my stress and feelings! I did not even know what feelings were.

My point in telling you about my history is that I now believe that stress, coupled with my unhealthy coping behavior, and poor nutrition led to the breakdown of my immune system, allowing the myriad changes that occur to enable cancer cells to go awry and set up house in my system, one more time. My emotional self is also responsible: the buried feelings, the lack of self-care, the being-there-for-all-but-Maria created the perfect setting for my two health opportunities. I refuse to say I have cancer. I will not give it any leverage. I am creating an environment in my body that is hostile to carcinoid. I will not run around looking for every possible cure, but I will use common sense and seek out what makes sense to me. If I am to die, I will not die an un-lived life, to quote the book by the same title.

Bill gifted me with a trip to Optimum Health Institute in Lemon Grove, CA in early May, 2011. I underwent a transformation that still has me reeling. I went to please him and lo and behold, I found Maria. I love her and I vow to stop polluting my body. I had taken better care of my car than I had done of myself, so I made a decision to stop eating sugar, stop caffeine, eat mostly raw food and no animals. I went inside myself and discovered the many feelings I still hold and which I had a chance to begin to release—fear, anger, sadness, grief, loss, anxiety, depression, self-righteousness, more fear. I cried more than I have in a lifetime. It is only the beginning and I know this new life is a process and not an event.

I have heroes in my life today, valiant people who have an amazing disposition, people like Susan "Sunny Susan" Anderson, my best friend Tina who believes in me as does Bill who knew to send me to OHI as he grew concerned about my negativity. My amazing and one-of-a-kind doctor-friends, Dr. Lally Pia, Dr. Martin Adler, Dr. P. E. D.A., the first person who reached out to me after reading one of my posts on a support group, J. S. the lady who started our local support group, Rosa with her Buddhist chants after her healing massage, along with many more friends who love me and whom I now allow to love me. My friend Marjie and her generous heart, my occasional walking partner and shopping buddy, and star cat sitter. I thank my support groups, on-line and group meetings. They share their knowledge, hope, and strength.

I will not be on my deathbed grasping at straws when my life comes to an end. By accepting that I could die and by resolving issues that needed to be addressed in my life has liberated more energy for healing! I will have lived a life filled with love, self-knowledge, a sense of humor, the love of friends and patients, colleagues, and pets (my beloved Jules and Medina in our house now; and Sammy and Milo who visit me in my dreams and who gave me unconditional love). My love of the wilderness: back-packing, hiking, rock-climbing, running—have all helped me become who I am and continue to do so.

I thank a Higher Power for allowing me to have my limitless life, for opening my eyes to a world of amazing friends and possibilities, staying open to change and growth.

I know that my spiritual path has a lot to do with how I accept this diagnosis. I have quit my job and volunteer with people who appreciate what I do, and I can set limits and have good boundaries. I believe in prayer, in my Shaman's love and healing. I believe in Jesus and the Buddha as my guides. As the poet Rumi said, "There are a thousand ways to kneel and kiss the earth". This whole experience has made me stronger, both emotionally and spiritually. I no longer fear cancer.

> *"Start by doing what's necessary; then do what's possible, and suddenly you are doing the impossible."*
> —St. Francis of Assisi

and

> *"Once the "what" is decided, the "how" always follows. We must not make the "how" an excuse for not facing and accepting the "what".*" Pearl S. Buck (one of my favorite writers)

I am grateful to all who stand with me, pray for me and always ask what they can do to help. I've learned how to forgive, an important skill in my growth. I've even forgiven my first oncologist, Dr. L., for treating me like a child and like a crazy person who was imagining her symptoms. I forgive him for looking for horses and not smelling the zebra, even if it was staring him in the face. I forgive his colleague, Dr. R. who called me at work, while I was seeing patients and, over the phone, abruptly announced I had "liver cancer" and had two months to live. I am so glad I fired you and Dr. N, (a second oncologist after my diagnosis). You would not listen. You would not look at articles from NET researchers, saying cursorily, "I have my own sources." Yes, you knew it all . . . and got it just exactly wrong. I let you go, I let you all go.

My current oncologist, Dr. E. Schmulbach is my ally and I thank him every day he goes to bat for me.

May I never forget the fragile bonds of cancer. Few without cancer appreciate the details, the visits to one another, the toll of treatment, the heavy conversations, the highs of good results, and the misery of bad news. I know now that the main challenges of being an oncologist are humanistic, not medical. Some do struggle to show their humanity, to let that humanity touch us. We form special bonds, as we communicate with each other, wrought through a common struggle, increasing over the course of years. We all fight carcinoid with knowledge and hope. I will not stop carrying the message as it was carried to me.

I want to be like Susan Anderson and L. W. to be there for others going through this dreadful disease, to welcome newcomers and help them understand their symptoms without overwhelming them with technical medical lingo. I appreciate J. M. and his amazing mind and ongoing quest to help all of us as we struggle with this cancer. I am so glad he is the leader of our support group in Walnut Creek, CA.

I still have fear, but it does not consume my every moment. I cope with the loss of my ability to run for miles; now I walk and appreciate that I can do that.

I appreciate my life more, its beauty and that of nature and all it gives me. I am very grateful to carcinoid for allowing me to see beyond the layers that make up my busyness, to reach into my core and my heart, to touch my Life. I am grateful to trust that I am loved. This is healing! While I do not expect a cure, I most definitely experience healing!

Dance out loud!

Beverly

Living with Carcinoid Cancer

I began experiencing abdominal pain in the summer of 2006 when I was 59 years old and working full time as an accounting manager. I was referred to a gastroenterologist for investigation of this symptom.

When all of my exams and tests came back normal, the doctor suggested one last test. I had to swallow a very large capsule which contained a camera. The camera took pictures as it passed through my digestive system and was to exit normally within 24 hrs. I have never been considered "normal" and, therefore, did not pass the camera. The pictures taken revealed tumors in my small intestine and the consensus was that I needed abdominal surgery, at which time they would surgically remove the lodged capsule. In September 2006, following surgery, I was informed that seven carcinoid tumors had been removed from my small intestine, and the good news was that it is a slow growing cancer.

Hurray, I was given the diagnosis of a "good kind of cancer!" My surgical report revealed that the surgeon had done a jejunal resection, resection of the mesentery and fifteen centimeters of small bowel.

I went along for three years feeling well, not experiencing any more symptoms. I was attending a carcinoid support group and wondering what I was doing there. Everyone else was having different problems, and I was feeling great. I asked if anyone ever gets cured with one surgery, and was told that it can happen. I felt guilty for going to the meetings and not having anything to contribute in the way of advice. I saw my oncologist every 6 months for follow-up and would get a CT of the abdomen and pelvis with oral and intravenous contrast. In May 2010, some changes appeared on the CT which included many abdominal tumors, as well as 2 tumors on the surface of my liver. I was told to see a specialist at UCLA, but that it could wait until I got back from Michigan in August.

In the meantime, a drug trial program became available. I started on the trial and would receive abdominal injections of interferon, 3 times a week. I started out with nausea after the injections and needed an anti-nausea pill for relief. When I traveled to Michigan by car, I was able to have a week off the drug, but had to start up again as soon as I got there. My oncologist in Michigan did not like me being on interferon and had me stop it. He also said he had a surgeon that could help me.

I had my second surgery on August 24th, 2010. I had carcinoid tumors removed from my omentum, 70 cm of right colon and distal small bowel, 3 lymph nodes, and removal of my left ovary. The liver tumors were deemed inoperable due to their location.

I have been living with diarrhea: ten to fifteen times per day since my surgery. Thus far, medications or diet have not lessened the number of stools I have. The diarrhea is especially severe after a large meal and I usually end up in the bathroom within five minutes of finishing a meal. This is followed by several more trips to the bathroom. I lost 40 pounds within the first 3 months of the onset of diarrhea and continue to lose weight. Some days I am extremely fatigued and try to drink Boost to replace lost nutrients in my body. I take Creon capsules before meals, which help break down fats and help my body retain some of the nutritional benefits of my meals.

My doctors and I are continuing to monitor the liver tumors, which have increased from two to four tumors and the first two have grown larger. In the meantime, another trial drug program is available in pill form: Sutent, which has some nasty side effects. I had decided not to go on this drug, because of its side effects. As it turns out, my insurance will not cover the cost of this drug. Sutent has been used for pancreatic cancer and was just recently approved by the FDA for carcinoid cancer.

In a nutshell, one is truly living on the edge, wondering and watching for this cancer to recur in another place. We not only fight the disease, but depression, the medications used to fight the cancer, and the insurance companies to get the treatments we need.

I tolerate my fight by making the crafts I enjoy so much. It occupies my time and my thoughts by means of concentration. I am a jewelry artist and sell my pieces at craft fairs, and a couple of consignment shops. I love to work with polymer clay to make unique, one of a kind jewelry pieces, as well as bead stringing, and bead weaving. I am now teaching a beginners bead weaving class!

I have a lot of things to occupy my mind. This is how I cope with my struggle with carcinoid cancer.

> *It is the heart, always, that sees before the head can see.*
> —*Thomas Carlyle*

Debbie L. Sanders

Miracles Do Happen!

Miracle #1, June 2006

After years and years of being told by local doctors that I had an "unseen" bleeding ulcer most likely caused by severe anxiety and "If I could just get a handle on kids and family life then I might start feeling better"—whatever! In the meantime, this "bleeding ulcer" was causing my hemoglobin level to drop as low as 6.75 combined with crazy pain prior to these bleeding episodes. I was also told I had IBS (irritable bowel syndrome) because of the severe bouts of diarrhea I was also having. I was sent to an allergist to find the cause of my extreme flushing. However, no allergy was found. After the last episode when my hemoglobin dropped to 6.75, my local doctors gave me blood and then hooked me up with an oncologist who began to treat me with IV infusions of iron and then later saline, only because I was complaining about how terrible I felt.

The lack of concern from local doctors prompted a "forced" trip by my mom to Mayo Clinic. When I got to Mayo in June 2006, I was exhausted, frustrated and I looked physically ill. My skin at this point was a waxy pale yellow color. After three very short days of tests Mayo Clinic confirmed that I indeed was not losing it and this was not an anxiety issue. Instead they diagnosed me with carcinoid cancer. The thought itself was devastating but also a relief! Now I had an answer and a plan of action and the comfort of knowing I was not nuts . . . let's count that as Miracle #1—My Mom's persistence and finding Mayo Clinic.

Miracle #2—August 2006

The doctors had scheduled my surgery for August 2006. My team of three of Mayo's top surgeons was to remove some identified tumors with the possibility of a liver resection (or, worse case scenario, perform a liver examination to consider a possible transplant). During this time I was never fearful, I was in complete peace. I knew I was sick, I knew something had to be done. I also knew God would be with me all the way. On the way to surgery I reached up to grab the hand of Jesus (in my mind anyway) and the old hymn, "Tis so sweet to trust in Jesus," came to my mind. I sang the only part I could remember, "Jesus, Jesus, precious Jesus! Oh, for grace to trust Him more!" For whatever reason, this was my song during that time. That day the hall to the surgery room was quite long and I never did have any warm fuzzy feelings, but I was at peace and was not afraid,: I knew Jesus was with me (even if I couldn't feel him). In the 8.5 hours of surgery the doctors removed my gallbladder to get to my liver—I guess you really don't need that? The surgeons then actually held my liver in their hands and ran an ultrasound over it, they found eleven tumors in my liver! The doctors decided that Radio Frequency Ablation was the best way to go, so they zapped them.

Yay! No liver resection or transplant required! They also removed twelve inches of my small intestine (the malignant primary tumor was found here). They also removed my appendix and some questionable lymph nodes. I was later told by my surgeon that they scraped hundreds of tiny grain-size tumors and removed the fatty veil covering my intestines. My Doctor told me, "they got anything they could see, feel, or touch", and I was as cancer free in those areas as possible. However because I had so many sand-like tumors, there was a good chance there could be more that he could not see. The only way to know for sure was to dissect me and he didn't suggest that at all. Yes, he had a sense of humor. But I was now good to go for quite a while! God's grace (No Fear), world class doctors and over twenty two tumors removed.

Miracle #3—Just hours after surgery

After that long surgery and the removal of these tumors I was actually up and walking that very day! Sore, unsteady on my feet, and feeling pain in every movement, I remember thinking "What did they do"? and "What was I thinking?" I couldn't believe they wanted me to be walking already! But, God was right there too. He sent me a beautiful, strong, orange-haired African American woman. Her spirit was firm, gentle, encouraging, but uncompromising, which is what I needed even if I didn't agree at the time. She praised the Lord out loud through the entire process. She gave me the strength and courage to walk and work through the pain. She was someone to guide me carefully through what I needed to do in spite of the pain and myself.

Miracle #4—Seven days after surgery

The Doctors released me to go home. I met with my consulting doctor at Mayo later that afternoon and he suggested that we stay the night just to be safe and because I was very tired. Since it was late in the day we agreed and waited. That night I started to bleed internally—by midnight, I was hemorrhaging. My family rushed me back to Mayo's emergency room and watched helplessly while the nurses started to put back all those crazy tubes. I remember crying, "Mommy, please don't let me die here!" I felt my life slipping away. I was so tired of hospitals. Within minutes, most of my surgical team was back at my side again. I was being scanned and having blood work done as they tried to find the source of the bleeding. Immediately they started a blood transfusion. Unfortunately I was passing the blood as rapidly as the new blood was going in. The human spirit is a funny thing: here I am sick with no energy and I keep singing that song "Jesus, Jesus, precious Jesus." Yes, this time I was scared and confused, but I had Jesus! God didn't let me go home and my family reacted quickly. It's great to be loved!

Miracle #5—The next morning

Even with all the scans and tests the doctors could not find the source of bleeding by early morning of the next day. At this time they thought the source of bleeding may be coming from somewhere within the intestines. With my poor husband by my side, I was passing bedpans full of blood and as strong as my husband is, this really got to him. The more I bled the more transfusions they gave me. Human blood does not smell pleasantly passing this way and there was a deathly stench that filled my room. One of my nurses was

101

young and fairly new. In the hurriedness of all that was going on, she spilled a bedpan of blood all over the floor in my room. She panicked, became very emotional, and, because of this, they sent her home. On her way out she encountered an older woman (maybe in her 70's) in the hall. The nurse told this woman that there was a very sick and possibly dying woman (me) across the hall from the patient's room where she was going to pray and asked if she would also pray for me. God was at work, setting the stage for miracle #6!

Miracle #6—

This older woman was my angel in yellow pants. She knocked on the door of my hospital room and asked if there was someone here who needed prayer. My husband's reply was, "If you believe in Jesus, then yes." She came into my room, blessed me with Holy water, placed three wooden crosses on my chest and prayed for what could have been only a few short minutes. Her prayer was interrupted by the head nurse who came in, asked the woman who she was and then, not so politely, asked her to leave. As she (my angel in yellow pants) began to leave, the nurse yelled to her "What did you spray in this room? Is that incense! What's that I smell?" The woman replied sweetly, "Maybe it's the Holy Spirit . . ." and then left.

The nurse then rushed me and my husband off to the operating room. They had my husband quickly sign all the paperwork for whatever they might have to do (the just-in-case stuff). Then doctors forewarned him that they may not be able to save me. In all this commotion I (in my mind) reached out to grab the hand of Jesus and again began to sing, "Jesus, Jesus, precious Jesus! Oh, for grace to trust Him more!" Jesus, Jesus, precious Jesus!" When I reached my hand for Jesus, I felt nothing and in the physical sense I never felt so alone. But spiritually in the depth of my soul I knew He was there with me even if I couldn't feel or see Him.

The first procedure was to be an MRI followed by a colonoscopy/endoscopy and then next would be surgery. After the first procedure the Doctors were baffled—there was now no bleeding found anywhere, it was as if it miraculously just stopped! They came out and told my husband the good news: the surgery was cancelled. The following morning my blood count was normal without having to have more transfusions and I was regaining strength. Just to be sure, the doctors repeated the lab work, and sure enough I was quickly on my way to normal! I was healed!

Miracle #7

The next day my angel in yellow pants came back to visit with me. We talked and I told her all that had happened after she had left and that I had thought maybe she was an angel. She assured me she was not an angel. She simply had come to pray for the nun across the hall when a distraught nurse asked her to pray for me. I told her, "That's what makes you an angel, your obedience to a request." She did give me her address and told me she was in her 80's. No one else saw this woman after that. I went to speak to the nun across the hall. I wanted to ask her to say thanks again to her friend. The nun's room was empty. She had been moved or had gone home. No one else remembers this woman except me, my husband, and the nurse, and no one else saw her the next day—except me. My Angel in Yellow Pants! Who needs wings when you have those awesome yellow pants!

The cool thing is that five years later, I am still here! I get to enjoy my family, friends and life! God now speaks louder through every day experiences, people and His word, all which I have a new appreciation for.

Blessings to all of you—Yes! God listens to prayers.

Surviving Carcinoid Cancer since 6/21/2006

> *Indeed we count them blessed who endure. You have heard of the perseverance of Job and seen the end intended by the Lord, that the Lord is very compassionate and merciful.*
> —James 5:11

B.F.J.

Life Imitates Career

At the time of my diagnosis I was a Registered Nurse Patient Advocate/Clinical Coordinator at a major medical center in Phoenix, Arizona. My role was to coordinate interventional treatments for persons with unresectable liver cancer. These treatments include Yttrium90 (Thera-Spheres® or SIR-Spheres®), hepatic radio-frequency ablations, cryo-ablations and chemotherapy embolizations. As always, it is not only about the physical being, but also the emotional and spiritual needs of the patient and their family and caregivers. I have done whatever is necessary to ensure that they receive the best care and an average work day could last as long as twelve to thirteen hours and that was okay. I have developed lifelong friends because of my role.

Our department had just purchased a CT scanner which could perform cardiac CT's. This would allow patients to have a specialized, non-invasive CT to look at the anatomy of heart arteries without an invasive procedure such as a cardiac catheterization. Part of any new program is the creation of processes to ensure that we give quality care. This included volunteers to have the procedure so the kinks (for lack of a better word) could be worked out. At the time I was 40 years old and a bit overweight so I thought I would volunteer. My rationale was if anything was positive, I would have the information and be motivated to make lifestyle changes. I also knew that our insurance would never cover this new procedure and this was an opportunity to have it done for free.

I was walking past some co-workers when I heard them talking about the process and informed them I wanted to enroll. I remember them telling me that the slots were filled and I would need to get special permission from my director, which I did.

I also received a lot of pushback from my peers. Comments such as "Why would you do this?" and "Don't you know by doing this you will have a hard time obtaining private health insurance?" (not a concern since I always plan to work for a big organization) to "Why do you want your coworkers in your business?"

The day of the CT scan, November 14, 2005, will forever live in my mind. I have horrible veins, so starting an IV was an ordeal. I'm also claustrophobic and had to have my head covered to even enter the scanner. Once the scan was complete I remember the room becoming silent. In retrospect this should have been an ominous sign. As I was dressing, a radiologist came into the room and explained that a 'spot' was found on my liver and she wanted me to have further work-up. I took this in stride as our livers have many spots and thanked her for letting me know. I then went back to work.

If it had not been for the perseverance of this radiologist I would have never followed up.

Next came dedicated imaging. Again, my veins are small, roll and lie deep in my skin. It took 2 RN's, a PT, and finally an interventional radiologist to locate a vein under fluoroscopy. I had the CT scan and wouldn't you know it, the machine went haywire and actually scanned my brain instead of my abdomen (yes, my brain is normal). By that time, I was mentally finished with this process. But, once again M.C. intervened, and we decided that I would have an MRI and a liver biopsy together.

As I have noted, I'm very claustrophobic. I know this as several years earlier, I volunteered for a cardiac research study I was working on and they had to take me out of the machine after five minutes. Therefore I had my MRI with sedation. They were able to see the area and decided on a biopsy. Even then I was not worried. As I was waiting between procedures, I worked and gave orders. This is hilarious, as I was under the influence of the sedation, and I have been told some of the orders I gave were downright crazy, but to me they made perfect sense.

Next came the waiting. Day One (no anxiety). Day Two (no anxiety). It was very hard not to just call pathology to get the results. (Hey, I work for the system and know everybody—smile). Day Three (98% calm). Day Four (90%). By this time everyone was starting to ask me about results, but I was still not too concerned as the hospital had been busy.

December 2nd, 2005, was and will forever be my D-Day. Hurricane Katrina had happened, and everyone including, Dr. Colombo were assisting the victims. Phoenix had become a hub for misplaced residents. She had approached me to help collect much-needed items. I had also ordered lunch for the staff and was in the process of passing it out to everyone when she came in the lounge and asked to speak to me. My first thought was about Katrina, but then the air felt different. I remember her taking me into a room with a stricken look on her face. The world tipped sideways, everything went into slow motion, and the air got heavier. I KNEW WHAT SHE WAS GOING TO SAY. "It's positive, you have cancer".

I screamed, "My son, my son, my son, he's only twelve years old!!" I remember the world turned a weird pink color as I began to cry. They asked if I wanted anyone to be called. My sister is a system director for our organization and our corporate office is located across the street. She literally came sliding across the street. Now I can laugh about it.

As you know, we feel that when we get a cancer diagnosis we are alone. However, I knew instinctively that that was not the case. One of the first people I called was a patient of mine who had been treated years ago and who had carcinoid. I remembered her positive attitude and her love of life and her knowledge of the disease process. I called M.B. and all at once our roles reversed, I was the patient and she was the mentor. I have been forever grateful to the love, knowledge, and support she gave and continues to give me.

I must tell you what happened to me on the day of my biopsy. One of my patients was going to receive a liver transplant. I was the first person she called once she was notified. We walked hand in hand to the pre-op area. I told her how a lesion was found and the plan of care. She was shocked and I reassured her that it would all work out. I explained how I would use this experience to be a better nurse/person for my patients and others who have gone through similar circumstances. She went on to have a successful transplant.

Back to my journey: After I was diagnosed I immediately went into survivor mode. I received a PET scan that day which was positive. I told the rest of my family, but the most difficult person I had to tell was my son. As a single parent, our relationship is close and it took every fiber in my body to remain calm and optimistic about my prognosis.

I was my surgeon's first appointment the following morning and we discussed options. I had worked with him for years in my capacity. It was deemed that I was a surgical candidate and was scheduled for the next morning. I was also scheduled for a prophylactic appendectomy and cholecystectomy. I didn't understand why at the time, but now I know that those are two places where carcinoid can originate. Also if Sandostatin* is needed, then it is better to not have a gallbladder. I also discussed a hysterectomy (this was a previously planned procedure for uterine fibroids) and learned a different surgeon was needed. Another sidebar,: since I knew a hysterectomy was planned, I had blood work drawn approximately one month earlier and all values were within range.

I went to work afterward and attempted to train someone to cover for me in the next six hours. I also went around my department to explain to everyone what was happening and to keep me in their prayers and thoughts.

The morning of surgery was a whirlwind. It was decided I needed a baseline OctreoScan™. I still had people to see and miles to go before I sleep, (a quote from Robert Frost's "Stopping by the Woods on a Snowy Evening").

I went to visit my patients who were in the hospital, including the young lady who was recovering nicely from her liver transplant. I had peers to visit across the hospital to get prayers and blessings. So much visiting until I was paged overhead and told to report immediately to pre-op (yes, they did that). I arrived winded but calm as I met the team who would prayerfully save my life.

Five hours later I was reborn. My carcinoid cancer was gone. I went back to work two months later and remain cancer free six years later. Initially, I would get a PET scan and an OctreoScan™ yearly therefore receiving imaging every six months. After my third year, my oncologist encouraged me to rely on octreotide only. I also have Chromogranin-A levels drawn. However, I did not have one done pre-surgery, so I lack a baseline. On year three, my octreotide scan was positive in my thyroid area, and I coerced my surgeon to remove part of my thyroid as a precaution, and fortunately it was negative.

I continue to be cancer-free six years later but I know that this illness can return. I feel blessed in all aspects of my life. I have seen my son become a man, was fortunate to take care of and love on my mom before she passed recently. My experience has made me a better Nurse Practitioner (recent graduate) to my patients and helps me understand their fears, hopes, and dreams as only someone with the disease can. I have become a mentor to others and a cancer advocate and speaker. I embrace new experiences, love all, enjoy the sunshine and rain and every breath I take. I take nothing for granted and count it all a gift.

Everything happens for a reason. Several years before the infamous CT scan, I was involved in an MRI cardiac research study (one of my roles), where volunteers were needed. This is how I found out I am claustrophobic and did not finish the scan. I often wonder, had I been able to complete the study, would the carcinoid been found then? Or, had I completed the MRI and it was negative, would I have done the CT study and it not been found? I am a Detroit native and moved to Arizona 13 years ago to be with family. Had I not moved would the tumor have been found? I was forty at the time and would have started menopause soon. I would have thought nothing of the flushing, mood or bowel changes that can happen with carcinoid patients and my outcome could/would have been different.

I know that the maxim, "It takes a village to raise a child" holds true for all of us. None of us should be or are in this alone. My health care team, my coworkers, friends, family and my son are what have kept me going. The members of my support groups keep me informed of the latest treatments and motivate me. Finally, people like the author of this book give us another outlet to share our story and encourage, motivate and educate the villagers as well as the children.

It's not what happens to you;
it's what you do with what happens to you.
—Aldous Huxley

Denise

My Carcinoid Journey

It all began the spring of 2009. I became very sick with bad diarrhea, throwing up and feeling really bad all over. I thought I had the flu which I rarely get in my life. I stayed home from work that day because I could not be far from the bathroom. I got up the next morning, had troubles right away but thought I would try to go to work anyway. I was going to be late because I had spent most of my time in the bathroom before leaving since I was still having diarrhea. I was running late for work so of course had to make up for it by going a little too fast. I got caught for speeding, tried to tell the patrolman I wasn't feeling well and I really wasn't at that point. I was sweating so bad and my heart was about to beat out of my chest, not from being scared but because I had also been having really weird heartbeats lately. He got done writing me a ticket, got back into the car and I

108

barely made it to work without having an accident: not a car accident, but a bad cramping stomach which made me feel like I was going to explode.

I continued to have these problems off and on all summer and had also become extremely tired. I would go out to my car at break, set a timer and take a nap. I couldn't stay awake at work. I would come home and sleep before getting supper. I had an appointment with my general physician and told her of my problems. She did some blood work and it came back that I was anemic. She put me on iron tablets to see if it would help. I also told her of the heart issue so she ordered a monitor to wear at night. That didn't show much but I still continued to have the rapid heartbeat that made my chest feel like it was going to explode.

My mother had just had surgery for an abdominal aneurysm and the doctor came out of surgery, looked at me and said you better get a scan because this is hereditary. I had been planning to anyway because it felt like every time I ate, I had rocks in my stomach and thought maybe I had one also. My mother had been living with her aneurysm for quite a while and they didn't do surgery until it got to a certain size. I told my husband after every meal, that there were lumps in my stomach and I felt so full. I could actually feel them.

I put off the test for a couple months, but something in my head said you better get it done now. I called for an appointment and it was set up for September, 2009.

I went in for a simple ultrasound on the abdominal area. As the nurse was scanning me she made me roll over and took some extra pictures. A lump came to my throat and I knew she had found something. At that time I only thought of an aneurysm. The technician couldn't say anything until the images were read by the radiologist.

Two days later as I was heading out the door to go to work, I got a phone call at 6:45 am, a call that changed my life forever. My general physician called and said you do not have an aneurysm but you do have a mass and it looks like cancer. I remember taking a deep breath and sitting down, asking her what to do. She said she would get things started for me to have a biopsy and CT scan. She asked to talk to my husband and as I sat there listening I felt fear creep in. When she hung up I headed to work, in shock as I recalled what I was just told. I still had to go to work and so I did, but drove slower that day. The twenty mile one way ride took longer to me than any other ride in my life. I didn't know what to think, how to feel and what to say. I got to work and my supervisor said, "Good morning. How are you?" I told her I didn't know how I was because of the phone call I had just gotten.

I was scheduled the next day for the biopsy and CT scan. I was terrified. I sat in my gown, waiting for them to come and take me to the room. When the doctor came in to explain what he was going to do I broke down crying. He was very kind and gentle. They wheeled me down to the room. I got on the table and an IV was placed in my arm for the dye. They did the CT scan first, then went in for the biopsy. What they wanted to do was not easy: the mass was lying between the stomach and liver. They inserted the needle but they couldn't get a sample as the needle kept bouncing off the mass and they never could get a good collection.

From that day on, it was all kinds of scans, from MRI's, brain scans, ovary scans, adrenal gland scans. You name it: I had it. Testing took the whole month of September. I continued to work every day trying to be normal but not knowing what "normal" was anymore.

The day finally came to meet with the oncologist to determine what they were dealing with. My husband went with me. We were in the waiting room with all the other people who were waiting to see a doctor or receive cancer treatment. I looked at them trying not to stare but wondered what their story was. Did they see the fear in my face? They had once been in my shoes also.

We were taken to a room with a sofa and some chairs. The oncologist came in and told me they found a mass. They thought it was lung cancer. The doctor quizzed me about my habits: Did I smoke or do I now? The answer was no. He said that where this mass was located was usually where smokers get cancer. I told him that I was a waitress at a truck stop for 15 years and smoking was allowed then, so when serving smokers, I had smoke blown in my face. Could that be the cause? After the visit, he wanted to examine me, so I was taken to the exam room. When he was done, another appointment was set up to visit with him about what he thought they were going to do.

We went back to the cancer center and met with the doctor. "You are young. We don't really know what kind it is, so we will hit you really hard with chemo", and he told me all the side effects and the schedule frequency. In my mind I did not feel right about any of this, and said I felt I needed a second opinion.

The doctor was actually okay with that. He asked where I wanted to go, and I told him my PPO would not work at Mayo, so I said Iowa City. He said he had an oncologist friend there and he would take care of the appointment and sending all my records to them.

By now it was October and I visited the oncologist at the University of Iowa City Oncology Clinic. The drive from my home is almost 3 hours. The doctor was a kind little man, with eyes that looked at me with sympathy. It made me feel like he was afraid to tell me what he was thinking. Not knowing what to think of what he was seeing from the scans, his answer was almost the same as my previous cancer center. I didn't like the answer. He said they needed more tests, different kinds of scans and more time. I drove back home feeling like my life was flashing before my eyes.

On my last visit with the Iowa City doctor, he scheduled me for a nuclear medicine imaging scan to detect if there were any more tumors or cancer cells in my body. The scan was a two day event. My arms were strapped to my body and a Velcro cover was placed over me so I felt like I was in a cocoon. I found it hard to breathe because it was tightly wrapped around me. The scan machine was very close to my body and the tip of my nose was very close to touching the machine. I had my whole body scanned.

Once done, I had to meet with the doctor. Technology has made things easier to do now so my test results were ready to view. The doctor was still unsure what type of cancer this was, saying that surgery was not an option. I looked at the computer with the picture of my tumor and asked, "Why not?" I said, "It looks like it should just be cut out." I wasn't convinced of his decision. He would get everything set up in Mason City, Iowa Cancer Center, since it was only 30 miles from my home, to start chemo and radiation. I left feeling like my world was closing in on me.

I was riding with my friend, both of us in silence. We were trying to absorb what was going to happen and what had happened. About 45 minutes later I got a call on my cell phone from the doctor. He said he had consulted with five other doctors and they did not agree with him. They said it was operable. He apologized with sincerity. So he made another appointment to come back and meet with the surgeon.

I returned yet again to meet with the surgeon, and he explained what he was going to do. I was set up for surgery in November 2009. I had known it in the back of my heart and God was speaking to me the whole time.

Surgery day arrived. My husband and friend took me to the hospital. I said goodbye to them and see you later. It didn't take long before I was being prepped. I kept calm by praying the whole time. The best part of the prep was when they did the epidural. I was so calm and relaxed. I could go back to that moment at any time in my head if I needed to calm down. Within minutes I was being wheeled into surgery. Drugs kicked in and I was happy as a lark. If I died on the operating table I would not have known it.

"Denise"—"Denise" . . . I kept hearing my name being said. I opened my eyes to a team of doctors hovering over me. I didn't know if I was alive or dreaming. When they knew I was awake enough they explained they had gotten it all. Surgery took five hours, they removed the tumor that was visible on all scans (but it wasn't the primary), removed nineteen lymph nodes, two sections of my small intestines, burned part of my liver out because it had metastasized there, took my right ovary and when they lifted out my stomach they found the primary inside the stomach so they removed it by taking three quarters of my stomach and rerouting my intestines.

I was cut open from top to bottom on my belly, with staples running all the way down and around my belly button. I had tubes running out of my nose, a catheter, and IVs. I am so glad for the medications that were given to me to keep me out of pain, but I couldn't tolerate them, so I told them to quit giving them to me and let me have Tylenol, Extra Strength. They gave it to me, and it worked just fine. They still were not sure of what kind of cancer I had, so they needed to study the tumors more before they could figure out a treatment. I became very depressed while in the hospital, three hours from home; no one could come to see me. It was so far to drive, so I was there the whole eight days without anyone. My husband had to work and he also farms, so I told him to not worry, but I sure wish there was someone there.

I wanted to come home but they were still trying to determine what the tumors were. Finally they came to me on about the sixth day after surgery and wanted permission to keep my tumors so they could study them. I signed the papers because if it can help another person with this same thing, then that would be great. They told me it was carcinoid, very rare, and what kind of treatment I would need. I got my first injection of Sandostatin˙ in the hospital and it hurt. What I didn't realize then that this was going to be what I now get every twenty one days for the rest of my life.

Finally on the eighth day after surgery the hospital staff came in and told me I am ready to go home. I called my husband and sister to come and get me. I was never so ready to get home and be with the people I loved. When he got there and saw me walking around, my husband was in shock. He was thinking I would be in bad shape, but truthfully I am a strong person, and I started walking the moment they told me to, to keep my strength up. When they came to get me, I rode in the wheel chair but slowly got in the vehicle, trying to be gentle on my stomach.

Once I got home, the challenge was where I was going to sleep. I couldn't climb the stairs and sleeping in a bed was not going to work. I was in too much pain for that. My recliner then became my best friend. I slept in that chair for five weeks.

About three days after being home, the area around my belly button became very red and inflamed. I was in the emergency room on Thanksgiving Day. The staples around my belly button were not healing and it was a mess. I received some antibiotics and was sent home. At my follow up appointment a few days later, they said it was not healing, so I had to pack it every day until it closed up. That area took five weeks to heal even though the staples had come out ten days after the surgery.

I learned fast what foods were not working for me. I had no idea what I really had even though they told me it was carcinoid. Nothing was said about much at all. I took matters into my own hands and started searching on the internet, learning more each day. I found others out there on Facebook and Twitter who share the same disease. What I have learned from all the others is so much more than what the doctors tell me. I continue to have labs and CT scans twice a year, then I visit with the oncologist and surgeon. My scans have come back all ok and labs as well. My liver enzymes were high but are all normal now. My weight has gone down 30 lbs. since the surgery. I recently started getting B12 shots because they took so much of my stomach that I don't absorb the B12 as well. I was getting so tired and tests showed that the levels were at the bottom compared to "normal" and what had been before.

Looking back, I now see all the symptoms but didn't have a clue what was going on with my body. My general doctor could not figure out what was wrong with me. I have had problems with unexplained diarrhea for a long time; couldn't be too far from a bathroom. I was heat intolerant. I didn't know what flushing was but thought it was hot flashes. My mood swings were terrible. I was so fatigued. I was in the hospital for ten days in 2007 for cellulitis in my leg. I became diabetic in 2008 and was diagnosed with carcinoid in 2009. My heart was beating so hard. Arthritis in my body has caused me to have two knee surgeries. I had so much swelling in my ankles and feet. I slept a lot and thought: if this is what getting older is, then I am not sure how much more I can take.

My life has changed so much. I want to do more than my body will let me, but I cannot, and pay for it if I do more than I should. If I overdo it, then my body aches all over, and I become so tired I can't keep going. I have a hard time eating because certain foods do not work for me anymore. I have blood sugar crashes quite often now since starting my regular medication. I still work full time but it makes me so tired. I have to work for the insurance. My husband is retired and on Medicare so I need the insurance. I am very thankful for insurance. I am very thankful they found this cancer and that I am alive today. The doctors told me if I had not been diagnosed when I was, then I would not be here today: I was at the end of my life then. I am thankful for the Sandostatin® but wish it did not have to cost so much.

I have tried to explain to the people I know about this type of cancer. I might look good which I am told all the time, but they do not know what I feel like on the inside. I continue to have days when I am in the bathroom more than I want to. My husband has been here for me, but doesn't understand when I am not feeling good. He

114

does not understabd what is wrong with me. I do not feel well for a couple days after I receive my medication. It feels like I have the flu. I have a son who doesn't want to learn much about it. I think he is afraid he might get it. My emotions are crazy some days. I work full time but am tired. I explain to others about the tiredness, but they don't really understand. Until someone has gone through this, they really don't take the time to learn nor do they want to. I am so happy to find support groups online so we can talk about what we are going through. I pray daily that I continue to have a job, so that I will have insurance. It scares me. I have so much more to learn. I am learning that even though we all have carcinoid, each case is different but yet we all share something. The people I have met online understand me and what I am feeling or going through. In contrast, the people I live with, work with, and love, do not understand. I am sad about that.

Dream as if you will live forever;
live as if you will die tomorrow!

—*James Dean*

Dennis Wood

I have kept up with "Sunny Susan" for several years but have never written to her nor met her. It has amazed me over my now 12 years since I was first diagnosed how little is known of or talked about the struggles with carcinoids.

I underwent all kinds of tests trying to discover the cause of my symptoms with everything from gallbladder, ulcers, and even stress being a suggested cause. Finally, in 2000, I was sent to a surgeon who opened up my abdomen to discover a small, 3 cm. growth in my small intestine. An inch and one-half was removed and three days later the surgeon announced that I had a carcinoid. He sent me to an oncologist for follow-up. The oncologist told me to come back and see him when I was sick. I "only" had a carcinoid (cancer-like) tumor.

I continued to follow up with a gastroenterologist. After two years my symptoms returned in 2002. Along with fresh biomarker labels, they confirmed something was happening again. The doctor said it was just scar tissue and not to be concerned. Four more years passed

(2006) and I was quite ill. Finally I returned to the surgeon who again opened me up and this time removed one and one-half feet of my small intestine. He removed two tumors measuring 3.5 cm and 5 cm with this second surgery.

The difficult part is that I now had tumors in my liver. The surgeon commented that the outside of my liver looked like someone had sprinkled pepper all over it: small "tumorlets".

I also developed two "very large" blood clots in the portal vein and I was given an anticoagulant to take. My life seemed close to ending.

At this point I saw an oncologist. This time, he said, I needed to be treated aggressively, but would not likely live but a few months. This took place in July 2006. I began what became 10 months of chemotherapy. The tumors in the liver shrank some and I enjoyed some good health with minimal symptoms, but chemo was taking its toll.

In 2007 the symptoms came back with a fury. By December I had to retire from being a pastor after almost 44 years. I was 61 years of age.

In December 2007 I was very weak, riddled with carcinoid and was given my first hepatic embolization. It brought great relief. The doctor said I could have one done every 6-12 months if I needed it.

I made it almost a year before the carcinoid syndrome became so severe that I needed something to be done soon. I put off the inevitable until March of 2009. This time a hepatic chemo embolization was done. I immediately began running daily fevers. Finally, by the month of May, I became severely jaundiced and went to the hospital. At the same time I was having a bad headache. The doctor took one look at me and sent me for a CT scan.

The scan revealed a brain bleed. I was put into ICU and within hours had a grand mal seizure. I had to be intubated and was in a coma for several days.

The fevers continued daily. The CT scan of my abdomen showed a 6 cm necrotic tumor in the liver. Where there had been two tumors, each 6 cm, there now was one necrotic tumor that then became abscessed. During an MRI of the abdomen I quit breathing again and was intubated. By this time I had become septic. I was once again admitted to the ICU in a coma.

Several days later I was out of the coma and back in a room. All together I spent 31 days straight in the hospital. I went home on antibiotics which my wife, my care-giver, administered intravenously. I still had fever constantly because of the abscess.

I was in and out of the hospital another 31 days during 2009 and 2010. I had from one to three tubes draining my liver abscess during this entire time. Blood counts were out of the normal range in almost every area.

I slowly began to improve.

The typical weakness and some of the symptoms of carcinoid syndrome continued, but much less in severity and occurrence. The last tube was removed in March of 2010. The fevers have completely stopped since then. The abscess was declared healed in October of 2010.

I am careful about my diet. I currently am on no medications. The last CT scan taken in October of 2011 shows a new tumor (7 mm) is now growing.

I daily thank God for life, my care-giver, my whole family, my support system, and am grateful for all. I will be 66 in March. I never expected to live this long. I am thankful for the opportunities to help other people with cancer, share with people about God's care, and encourage people with a weekly devotional on my blog site:

www.dgtheencourager.blogpot.com

God has been good to allow me to continue with a ministry of writing and speaking.

I learned that a highly developed purpose and the will to live
are among the prime raw materials of human existence. I
became convinced that these materials may well represent the
most potent force within human reach.
—Norman Cousins

Danica C

I guess my story begins in January 2006 (I think). I had fired my most recent doctor and was going in to see a new one. At this point I had seen seven doctors in four years and I was ready to give up. Before I walked into this new doctor's office I had decided this would be the last one. When she came into the office and before she could say anything, I told her, "I have seen seven doctors in the past four years and all of them have told me there is nothing wrong with me and it was all in my head. If you don't want a challenge I will walk out of here and you will never see me again."

This doctor sat down and spent the next 45 minutes with me and came up with a plan. First she ran blood work. More blood work and labs than I had ever had before. When most of that came back normal she started looking elsewhere. She sent me to specialist after specialist. Nothing . . . She called me one day and told me to go get a chest x-ray as she thought maybe I had inflammation around the heart. Before I even got home that day she called me on my cell phone and told me she wanted to see me in her office the next day. She couldn't say anything over the phone.

When I went to her office, she told me they saw a mass in my right lung and she was sending me to a pulmonologist to have it biopsied. Things went really fast after that. When I had the biopsy done I ended up having to stay overnight because they collapsed my lung.

Then I waited for results. A few weeks later I got a phone call from the pulmonologist while I was working. He began by telling me they figured out what it was. OK . . . fine . . . then he went on to say, "Well, you have cancer. It's called carcinoid. It's a two centimeter tumor in your lung." He said he didn't know that much about it, but he gave me the spelling and told me to look it up. REALLY!! I was stunned and a little freaked out. He told me this over the phone while I was working.

I walked into my boss's office, told her and she sent me home for the day. I got to the car and called my husband. He was a little more than upset that I was: 1) told over the phone and, 2) while I was working. My husband told me to stay there and that he was coming to get me. I remember almost nothing of the next few days. I was stunned and overwhelmed. Other than my husband I had no one to talk to and no one called.

I did what I was told and researched it. I found out a whole lot of information and when I went in to see the oncologist, I showed him my research and he wasn't as impressed as I thought he would be. He outright yelled at me for trying to do his job. I was stunned and so was my husband who looked as though he was going to punch out the doctor. I didn't blame him. Then he told me I had to have surgery or I would die. He said he was referring me to a surgeon. Then he got up and walked out. My husband and I were left there just looking at one another. I don't think we spoke all the way home. Not because we were mad at each other, but because we were outright stunned.

There was one thing I had done a few months before all of this happened and I'm sure happy that I did. To this day I still have no idea why I did it. An AFLAC representative came in to our office selling insurance and I ended up getting a cancer policy that day. I just had a very strong feeling I needed to do this. Of course my husband thought I was off my rocker, but it was only a few dollars a paycheck. I almost stopped it. I didn't know at the time that I would actually need and use it.

I don't remember much between the times of seeing the outraged oncologist until I met with the surgeon. I do however remember that morning when we were going to see the surgeon. I told M. that morning that if I did not like the surgeon I would walk out and not return. When he walked into the room I was put at ease. He was the kindest person and listened to me. I felt very good about all of it when we walked out.

The next few weeks and months were filled with tests and scans. I went in for surgery on May 31, 2006. Everything seemed to go according to plan. The surgeon went in and removed the lower lobe of my right lung via thoracotomy. Towards the end of my surgery something went wrong and the anesthesia started to pool in my hand, and I went into crisis. The nurse went out to talk to my mom and my husband, mentioning something to that effect, and when she realized no one had mentioned it before, she clammed up. To this day we still don't know what happened. I was wheeled into recovery and I was in ICU for two days. It took twelve hours for me to come around after surgery. No one could or would explain why or what happened.

I spent the next week in the hospital. I went back in to the oncologist a few weeks later and he pronounced me cured. That was not the end of it but rather the beginning.

I went back to work after a few months, but became very sick again within a few weeks. I returned to my Dr.'s office and she sent me over to the hospital for emergency gallbladder surgery. I was in the hospital for a few days before I could have the surgery as my potassium was very low. I had to have potassium infusions before they could do my surgery. It took two days before they could stabilize me enough to have surgery. I went into carcinoid crisis during surgery again because they did not have the octreotide drip on hand! I eventually recovered from this set back and returned to work again.

Later that year in late December, I returned home from a work Christmas party to my phone ringing. I thought it was a strange time for my doctor's office to be calling me. After all, it was after 6 pm. The nurse on the phone was telling me I had to come in right away. I had been in the office the day prior and had routine blood work done. I thought it was routine. This nurse went on to tell me that because of my condition it was urgent I go in for a potassium infusion or I could go into cardiac arrest. I asked her what she meant by "my condition?" She said, "Well you know you are pregnant right?" I told her she was crazy because they told me I would not be able to get pregnant and I went on to tell her she had the wrong person. I am certain it took her ten minutes to convince me she did have the right person. I was in shock and terrified. In the weeks prior I had been through lots of testing in the nuclear medicine department. Not only that but I had had CTs, MRIs and x-rays. I could only imagine what all this must have done to the life growing inside me.

I recalled having had an octreotide scan two weeks prior and they had seen something pop up on the test that kind of surprised them. In the report it stated that there was a hot spot near or in the uterus and I needed to see my OB/GYN for follow up. At that point my doctor had been contacted and asked me to go in for blood work. I thought it was routine, like I said. Turned out she ran a pregnancy test and that little hot spot they saw on the scan was my little P.!

Once again my husband and I were completely overwhelmed with doctor appointments. Early on we were advised to terminate the pregnancy because they had no idea what all the radiation might have done to the baby. One of my first appointments we went to was a parade of doctors coming in and out of the office. I think all in all there were twelve I saw that day. I felt like an experiment or some kind of carnival freak. I even had more than one doctor yell at me for being so careless and getting pregnant in the first place. It was not like I meant for that to happen, after all, we were using birth control.

The pregnancy was compounded with difficulties because of the fact I was still recovering from lung surgery. It was a miserable eight months. I was so sick most of the time. I was suffering from carcinoid syndrome and was constantly in the doctor's office getting infusions of potassium and IV fluids because of the persistent diarrhea and vomiting I was now having.

I had hoped to deliver P. naturally, but because of my condition and because they really did not understand how my body would respond to the stress of natural childbirth, they decided to do a C-section. The surgery did not go as planned, because at the time, they had considered me cured and did not have an octreotide drip on hand. My blood pressure dropped and they had to call for a crash cart. Things turned out OK after that and my little P. was born. She was very small at 5 pounds 10 ounces and she was a little early at 34 weeks gestation.

It took another year of suffering with carcinoid syndrome symptoms before I convinced my doctor to do a 5-HIAA test and they could see something was not right. I was put on sub-Q injections of octreotide and I did this myself for another year. I did these until we moved in 2009 when I was finally put on the Sandostatin LAR° injections.

I have never really stopped to think about my diagnosis. As far as coping, I don't really. I don't let myself get stuck in my head thinking about it. I take everything day by day. I have a hard time looking at myself as being sick. I have always taken care of everyone else and have always been the strong one. I have hidden from everyone how much I really suffer with all of this. I have always played everything down as to not let anyone really know what is going on. I don't think even our families really understand. Recently it has become difficult to hide it and I have had to come to terms with it all. I still don't ask for help, and I think that bothers people (including my husband), but

I am learning slowly. I have never found it easy to deal with my own problems.

My explanation to myself has been that because they have not found any more tumors maybe it is not so bad. I know this is not true because I live with the symptoms of the syndrome every day. Sometimes it is easier not to think about it and just push it aside and take care of my family.

Up until 2011, it was easier to just not say much to people. I was able to take care of most things on my own. Around November 2012, I started to get very ill once again. I was hospitalized with what they called an ileus, where my insides just shut down. I had to have an NG tube put into my body for a few days. What a nightmare that winter was. I was in and out of the hospital three different times and have never quite been the same since. I now have to rely on people more. I have not been able to drive now for a couple of years due to vision problems, as well as the fact that my reflexes, because of a movement disorder, are not what they should be. I was advised not to drive at all!

This has completely changed our lives. It makes it very difficult for me to do what I really want to and I get very frustrated at times. I know it is hard on my husband as he is in school to get his degree to make things better for us. He tries to spend his time between trying to make things better for us and his outside issues. He takes care of me and helps with P., our youngest, who is now five. S., our 17 year old, is almost grown and my husband runs her around where she needs to be. He also helps with most of the housework. I feel bad because I used to do most of the housework and took care of our girls. Now that I am unable to do any of this, I try to do what I can to help out.

Our youngest is a huge challenge for us as she was diagnosed on the autism spectrum, is epileptic and has moderate hypotonia (previously known as "floppy baby syndrome".) It is characterized by abnormal and reduced muscle tone and muscle weakness. She was born fairly small and has had challenges since birth. At 18 months of age, she had two grand mal seizures and this changed everything. She is now 5 and thriving in kindergarten. She still has a long road ahead of her with these issues, but she has a good chance at a really good life with a lot of support.

My husband and I have no real plans. I think we have not wanted to see it or really face it head on. We have started talking more about it recently and really should start making some sort of plans. Just talking about our problems right now is a good start (I think). I know I still have a little time left (or so I hope, as no one ever really knows how much time they really have).

I have gotten really good at not facing my future. It is difficult for anyone, but when you have a special needs child who will need support most of her life, it is twice as hard. I know there will be many who will be able to step in for me and my husband will be there for her as will her sister. However, as a mom, I want to be there for both my girls.

As I said before, we do not know how much time we have left on this earth. We just have to do the best we can with what we have. I hope it will be enough and hope my girls and my husband always know that no matter what happens, I love them with all of my heart.

At this time, since writing my initial story, I am on TPN as I wait for doctors to find out what is causing me to have abdominal pain, nausea, vomiting, and inflammation around my duodenum. I have pain with eating, but this is improving. I am feeling very depressed and have lost a lot of confidence in my medical providers.

I have many people who love me, both family and friends and they, together with my belief in God, are keeping me going.

Life can only be understood backwards;
but it must be lived forwards.
—Soren Kierkegaard

Nancy

It all started one weekend in May 2008. I was at home when all of a sudden, I got the worst case of diarrhea I'd ever had in my life. I went through my clothes, used napkins and towels, but nothing could hold it back. It gave no warning at all that I can recall. It would hit me every so many hours. Nothing I ate would prevent it. I ended up in my local ER where they ran a few tests. I thought I had food poisoning, as there had been a tomato salmonella outbreak. I got tested for the six most common things that can make you have diarrhea. They discovered I had one of the worst kidney/bladder infections the ER doctors had ever seen. Had I not come in and been admitted, they said that I would have had 24 hours to live.

During this time I was admitted for 1½ days and thought that this infection explained the on-and off pain I had been having to the left of my belly button. They gave me five shots of morphine, which hardly killed the pain I was experiencing. They also performed a CT scan and everyone failed to notice that I had a small bowel obstruction!

I went home for a few weeks, and every so often the pain on the left side of the belly button would return. The pain got so bad that I couldn't eat or drink without throwing up. Even water would come back up within the hour. I would take medicine and it didn't even have the chance to dissolve in my system.

Back to the emergency room I went. I was given IV pain meds and sent home with instructions to come back if it wasn't any better. I came back. I was throwing up in the ER with pain so bad that I was doubled over. It was the 4th of July holiday. Of course there were no surgeons available. I got so fed up. I visited four different hospitals in one night. By the end of the night I was back to hospital number one.

They decided to give me contrast and check to see what was going on. After 4 hours, nothing; after 24 hours hardly anything showed up in the colon. Forty-eight hours later, they decided to do exploratory surgery. I was prepped, ready for surgery and the doctor who was supposed to do the surgery got severely ill and called it off. I had to wait until the following day for the operation. I woke up post-surgery, hallucinating in the ICU, having never even met my surgeon. An unknown person walked into my room and told me that I had cancer, but they didn't know what kind it was. They had never seen this before, but told me I had less than six months to live. Then they came back and said, "No, you don't have pancreatic cancer, rather you have ovarian." After further tests were performed, they told me, "No, you don't have that either." Oh goody, I have cancer and no one has seen this before. I began to hope this all would turn out to be a lie. They sent the tissue to an out-of-state pathology center to be analyzed. The pathology results came back as a typical mid-gut carcinoid.

They started me on sub-Q shots of octreotide in the hospital every eight hours. They made me so ill that I had to take Benadryl and anti-nausea medication a half hour before getting the shots. I spent the entire month of July 2008 in the hospital, followed by ten days in a Rehab facility.

Then I was off to southern California for a second opinion and to begin learning. While I was waiting for my appointment in the glass-wrapped lobby of the medical center, I got ill again. I had a three-hour consultation on the ins and outs of this rare cancer. I was admitted to the regular hospital with what turned out to be four blood clots: two in the right leg, and one in each lung. I began to think that if the cancer didn't kill me, these blood clots would. I spent twelve days in Los Angeles. I had an endoscopy, an MRI, and swallowed a pill camera to check my colon.

Since that first operation, my bio-markers started rising. Soon I was off to see an oncological Ob/Gyn doctor for a possible hysterectomy. I took a year and half to make the decision to proceed with that and debulking surgery at the same time. I spent nine days in the hospital after that surgery because I kept throwing up. The blood work showed my potassium and magnesium levels were dangerously low.

It took about one year for me to recover from that surgery and feel back to normal once again. I started out with Sandostatin LAR° 20 mg. very month. When that didn't help and I was continuing to have carcinoid syndrome, my dosage was increased to 30 mg. LAR every month. When that didn't help, my dosage was increased to 30 mg. every three weeks.

I have tried to quit Sandostatin LAR° five times because of the side effects I experience and have been off of it now since early 2012. My biomarkers are once again starting to climb. I rarely flush and have no diarrhea. I don't know what the future will bring.

I lost close to 60 pounds during my stays in the hospital and barely ate for two to three months. I now consume just about anything and have gained back all my weight, which is not good.

I feel well but still get tired. Living in Las Vegas with the 110 degree plus days of summer makes it harder to cope some days. I had gone to a local gym until I developed cellulitis in my right leg; therefore, I have had to quit exercising for now.

I've learned to get the results of all my blood work and scans and keep my own set of copies. I file these by year so if I have an issue, I can refer to my own copy. I feel it is very important to do this. You have to be your own advocate because no one else will do it for you. Unless your friends or relatives are in the medical field and can help you sort out the insurance and medical mess, the challenges this creates for you and your family feel overwhelming.

I really feel that anyone with carcinoid needs to stay connected either to a local group or on the internet. Don't be afraid to reach out for help, because we don't judge you. We bring our issues to the table so we can learn from each other. Please take the step and reach out to others who can understand where you are coming from. Even if your family members are not supportive, do it for yourself and your mental health. I take it day-to-day and try not to think long term.

The hardest thing about this cancer is family members who are in denial. They don't want you to talk about it or discuss it, never ask how you are doing, and rarely or never call. Then there are your friends and fellow church members who say, "You look so well". They don't understand the drugs that give you brain fog and make you even more fatigued. They don't see that you get tired after years of going to every doctor imaginable for this issue and that issue, all the blood work, shots, poking and prodding that goes on week by week, month by month, year in and year out. They are blind to even the insurance issues that we have to deal with. Then there are the Social Security offices that determine that you're not sick enough and all you need is a hysterectomy and you'll be fine. Denied, knowing you will probably never hold down a full-time job, just because they say you are a cancer patient and you're too expensive to deal with. Others who say, "You need to eat healthier or lose weight", and think that will cure you in a few months. It does help with daily living, but it is not a cure. True cures will come from God himself and no one else.

For over 1½ years now I have had no major health insurance. This means no scans, no hospitalization, no surgery, and no major medical treatments unless I pay for them out of pocket. I do have a minor health insurance policy that provides benefits only for doctor visits, office procedures, and the shots I need, including my B12 shots and iron transfusions. This policy is available to me on a year-to-year basis, and each year it is amended. Once January comes around, I have no idea what will be happening in this situation.

Your doctors need to be able to talk to one another. If not, then change doctors. Don't take "No" for an answer. I have kept all my doctors whom I met four years ago and rely on a lot.

I co-launched the NETs/Carcinoid Cancer group here in southern Nevada and found many others who are suffering from this disease. It has helped me a lot with my coping issues, knowing, day or night, I have good friends to turn to.

I rarely think about my cancer and try each and every day to move forward with God's help and the backing of my church, who prays for my healing and for all cancer patients. I re-dedicated my life back to the Lord in December 2008 and have grown daily by reading the word of God. I pray daily for a medical breakthrough for those suffering with carcinoid cancer and hope you will do so also.

Anonymous

I am 13 ways tough!

I was diagnosed in January 1999 when a routine colonoscopy revealed a tumor at my ileocecal valve. Pathology of the tissue revealed it was carcinoid. A follow up CT scan showed lesions in my liver. Several were about 2 cm and more tiny ones were seen as well. A right hemicolectomy was done removing the primary and taking a wedge biopsy of my liver. The pathology showed that it was carcinoid metastases for sure. If I had known then what I know now I would have tried to have the liver transplant surgeon there cherry-pick some of the spots out of my liver while I was open instead of just doing the wedge biopsy.

I went to the Mayo Clinic in Rochester, Minnesota for a second opinion. My planned out schedule said I was to see the reputed carcinoid expert there. I didn't see him but had an MRI and saw a very pleasant and knowledgeable young South American woman M.D. who told me about Sandostatin® and chemoembolization. She explained why chemotherapy usually was not helpful to typical carcinoid patients because of the slow-growing cells being resistant. So I was treated in Iowa (where I live) by a bright oncologist who was not a carcinoid specialist. I started on Sandostatin® subcutaneous shots and was on interferon for about a month. On interferon, I was fatigued and sort of depressed and "headachy". (I think now the dose was too large, and I would not hesitate to try it again if my tumors seem to be growing because there were no lasting ill effects). I felt great immediately after stopping interferon. That oncologist moved away and I saw another one who is a very smart, very sweet man, who does not pretend to be a carcinoid guru but he is humble and willing to listen and learn, and later that year, a physician who focuses on carcinoid came to Iowa.

As for symptoms, I had had bouts of unexplained diarrhea going back as far as 1974. They would start with what was very much like the 24 hour "ick" that goes around sometimes, although I wouldn't feel sick, just have the runs very badly. To be grossly graphic, I might eat some lettuce or spinach and recognize it in the toilet a half hour later, after great rumbling noises from my intestines. My internist would do stool cultures and blood tests and find nothing wrong. I'd get a prescription for an anti-diarrheal and the episode would finally pass. I have had problems with anxiety my whole life and I think my doctor and I kind of thought that this was a manifestation of that, although he was a wise and thoughtful man and did not tell me it was in my head. I probably suggested anxiety myself, and, since he found no physical ill other than the diarrhea, he saw that as a possibility.

I had colonoscopies every several years because both my parents had colon cancer (not carcinoid) and my grandfather had rectal cancer. When my internist and I learned of the carcinoid finding, I asked, "Well, how are your other carcinoid patients doing"? He said, "You're my first." At the time of my diagnosis, I was started on blood pressure medication and had some very scary readings a few times. They were in the 200+/100+ range. A new internist has had that nicely under control for some time now. (I didn't fire the old internist, he moved to another hospital).

I tried Sandostatin LAR˚ for several months but think that the sub-q product works better for me. There seem to be so many complaints about somebody not administering it correctly. I only complained of a sore lump once when a different nurse did it but I still like sub-q better. I think I have more control with it. I'd try the pump except I don't like fussing over technical things; my phone and computer and C-PAP machine and hearing aids are enough.

I recently had my twice-yearly MRI and it was again called "stable disease". My big complaints are with joint/muscle/whatever, that makes my back, hips, shins, and feet hurt and recently my neck too. I fear metastases, but my doctors seem to think osteoarthritis is the explanation. I really do not like to attribute most everything that ails us to carcinoid. I am waiting for somebody to think their hangnails are a carcinoid phenomenon. I just don't like to give this darn disease credit or blame for everything.

How do I cope? Well, I try to eat nutritious foods such as oatmeal, fruit, vegetables, fish, and skim milk. I do not eat anything out of the ordinary except soy milk (chocolate!). I make myself exercise almost every day on the NuStep° (treadmill hurts as I can't walk distances without "ouchies"). I live at a retirement community in an independent apartment. Since I have no relatives closer than cousins and no spouse or children, I thought after my diagnosis that I should move here. It was a wise move, although I think it is too bad that age groups are lumped together. Generations are getting more mixed with the economic situation making people live with more extended family members at times here recently.

I have always been kind of a skeptic about a lot of things (never really believed in Santa Claus, and certainly not in the tooth fairy) so spiritual and religious things have not been a great comfort to me. I try sometimes but still doubt. I have lots of nice acquaintances here. My all-time favorite friends (those still alive: I'm 79) live in Maine and Alaska so my support from them is by phone.

It takes courage to live in a cancer-ridden body.

BE YOURSELF—ALWAYS!

Bill Manewal

Caregiving in the Context of Life

There's a documentary film titled: "Crazy, Sexy Cancer." Uh, yeah, sometimes. But mostly, cancer sucks.

"Don't mistake that stool sample in the fridge for hummus."

Stuff like that. Like the fact that as a child, nobody in my proper Protestant family ever farted. I'm sure they must have passed gas, but they never farted. Now my partner does so, continuously and explosively, and we've learned to laugh about the "prize winners." It's no contest: she wins.

I've actually put off writing my experience as a caregiver and I didn't know exactly why until last night, when I awakened with a flash of insight: I was afraid to tell the truth to my partner.

I'm a guy. The "patient" and my beloved partner is a woman. When a woman is scared, the guy is supposed to take care of her, comfort her.

My partner's personality is much more expressive emotionally than mine. She can range from giddy child-like delight to the depths of depression with thoughts of suicide. The emotional storms riding the deep-water currents of hormones released by neuroendocrine tumors don't help the process. The phrase "carcinoid rage" seems about right sometimes.

The one emotion that takes charge much of the time is a crippling force in her life, and therefore in our lives, is fear and its dysfunctional attendants: anxiety, hopelessness, helplessness, depression.

Fear of what? How about death for starters. Or being paralyzed from bone mets. Or incontinence. Or bloating, with yellow eyeballs, from a failing liver. Pain. Intractable and chronic pain. Or being so weak that walking is simply not worth it. So far, only the pain has presented itself in real time.

In the face of all of her fear, which sweeps over her in lunar-like cycles and is strongly correlated to whatever test or procedure is next on the agenda, I feel that I must be, shall be, cannot be other than: stalwart. Stoic. Encouraging. Offering hope. I cannot admit any fear at all. I tried expressing my feelings one time, and it freaked her out. Freaking out is the last thing someone with a weakened immune system needs. You see, I'm a nurse, so I really do know what stress can do to our body/mind/spirit: It kills us.

So I've learned to talk about my fear with people other than my partner. It works.

So what, you might be asking, does all this do to a relationship? It can, of course, kill it. We've all heard stories of spouses bailing. If not physically leaving, then emotionally, either with silence, overeating, computer addictions, overworking, cheating, alcohol, gambling . . . you name it.

I resent cancer's intrusion into our lives. I resent being chained to a medical center and the interminable tests and waves of uncertainty and fear and just plain medical and bureaucratic ineptness we have to subject our lives to. Sometimes I just want to whine. Or yell. Pitch a fit about having to be so much of a researcher and an advocate in the face of an incompetent medical system. But I can't: my partner is sick even though she's also healthy and living right now, just across the same room. So I take it elsewhere and that seems appropriate.

When my partner is really feeling sorry for herself, she sometimes says things, like, "You should just move on. Find someone else. Someone who's not sick, not dying."

I have requested she not say this. She promises and then it comes around again. Frankly it pisses me off, because it casts my commitment to her and to our relationship in a very shallow light.

In sickness and in health, until death do us part. And, in my view, not even death will part love. Love is all there is. It may not be all you need, but it is all there is.

Look, we're all gonna die. None of us makes it out alive. As the bumper sticker says: "100 YEARS . . . ALL NEW PEOPLE."

So the question becomes, what are we going to DO about it? Commitment isn't a word: it's an act. In my experience, about 99.9% of us North Americans relate to this inevitable destination of life with at least 100% denial. I suspect that in Africa or Afghanistan where death is more of a daily companion, the people have a much different and more accepting relationship to dying, to living in the face of death.

In spite of such absurd sticking-head-in-sand behavior, or maybe because of it, most of the world's spiritual teachers have told us to live most fully, we must be fully aware of the end of our lives. Poetically, I remember Carlos Castaneda's character Don Juan Matus telling him:

> *How can anyone feel so important when we know that death is stalking us? The thing to do when you are impatient is turn to your left and ask advice from your death. An immense amount of pettiness is dropped if your death makes a gesture to you, or if you catch a glimpse of it, or if you just have the feeling that your companion is there watching you.*

Better get used to it. Sure, we can rage against it, accept it, learn from it, cry about it. But in the end, none of that makes any damned difference as far as not dying. What is affected: our present lives.

I choose my partner. Every day. I choose to see her as living while she's dying, just like every one of the rest of us. On her good days, she sees that too. I pay attention to her fear: not so much to what she's afraid about, because almost always it's not happening now or what is happening now doesn't mean what she's afraid it means. I try to honor her fear and encourage her to catch herself from making up stories that scare her out of her strength.

Cancer changes lives and relationships. The biggest lesson I've gotten is that it forces me to accept what is. "Survive" means to "live through." I'm going to live through this process because it is what's so. To do so with some perspective, humor, skill, grace, laughter, tears, and lots of love is what I aim for, and sometimes achieve. When I fail, I apologize.

The biggest hazard in a caregiving relationship, aside from the temptations to bail or check out, is to become burnt out as a caregiver. We must take care of ourselves, by setting limits as to what we are willing and not willing to do, by taking time to re-create our true selves through meditation, retreat, or things that are just plain fun. If *we* don't get our needs met, we can't possibly be of use to others: compassion fatigue sets in and it's horrible stepsister: resentment of other. I am learning the functional approach of communicating my feelings and my boundaries with my partner, *before* the resentment builds. Sometimes I have to remind her that my boundaries are necessary for my mental health, and are not a negative reflection on her or the fact that she has a long-term, mysterious, and often debilitating disease.

> *Though the mills of God grind slowly, yet they grind exceeding fine.*
> *Though with patience He stands waiting, with exactness, all He grinds.*

I've come to figure out that we are here to be ground up, to be composted, transmuted, one way or another. My resistance to this immensely powerful, awesome inevitable process causes immense suffering. But when I embrace the flame of my attachments being burned, even by accepting the spiritual challenges of enduring the edgy process of cancer, I find myself living free. Then I'm able, through perspective and humor and love, to find ways our relationship can be about something other than "All Cancer All The Time." We can change channels. Cancer is not wonderful, but the life it's an integral part of, can be glorious. And often is.

> *Teach us to care and not to care*
> *Teach us to sit still.*
>
> T.S. Eliot

Amy

My Personal Survivor Story with Neuroendocrine Cancer

The words, "you have cancer" are probably three of the most profound words I have heard in my life. The words knock the wind out of you—drop you to your knees. I remember bawling in my mom's arms telling her "I don't want to die. I am too young. I have two babies." At the time I had three and four year old boys.

I was thirty-five years old. I had had strange symptoms for over two years, probably much longer—fevers, unbearable pain in the upper right side of my stomach, overall exhaustion and a gut feeling of something not being right. I went to urgent care clinic nine times over the course of two years. At age thirty five, I still had not picked an internist! I finally landed in the emergency room following a persistent fever that wouldn't break. They sent me home after filling me with fluids with no explanation. "What about appendicitis," I asked the on-call doctor. "Listen, I saw the way you walked in here, if you had appendicitis, you would need to be wheeled in in a wheel chair, screaming at the top of your lungs in pain." This was his reply to my plea for understanding what I was being treated for.

Thankfully, my mother doesn't take no for an answer! Frustrated, she drove me that Monday morning to my gynecologist. Having had two small boys, she was the only doctor I had at the time! My mother insisted on a CT scan. Based on the scan, I was in laparoscopic surgery the next morning. "Your appendix looks odd" was the reasoning.

133

That afternoon, we got a call from my surgeon, "there was a 2.1 cm tumor in the appendix but I have done hundreds of surgeries and it doesn't look like cancer, but the specimen will be sent to pathology. I will call you with the results in a few days."

That night, I began an obsessive thinking pattern that would continue off and on over the next two years. I stayed up well into the morning googling appendix growths, 2.1 cm tumor, severe pain in abdomen, fevers, appendicitis. I searched for anything that would remotely sound like what I had been told was wrong with me. The next morning I told my husband. I found information on two cancers of the appendix, carcinoid cancer and something called PMP Appendix Cancer. I kept going back to the calming words of Dr. Stricheartz, my surgeon, "I have seen many tumors and this tumor doesn't look like cancer." For some reason, those words weren't enough to ease my growing anxiety.

Three days later, my mom and I were in the kitchen when the phone rang. It was my gynecologist, Dr. Truneh. He asked if I was alone. My stomach sank. I informed him that my mother was with me. He told me the results of my pathology were back and wanted to know if I wanted my mother to listen in on speaker mode.

My hands began to shake and my face felt warm. As I pressed the speaker button, my mom looked at me with fear in her eyes and tightly grabbed my hand.

Dr. Truneh told me, "Amy, sweetie, I am sorry, it is cancer. It is carcinoid cancer and it's very rare. We made an appointment for you to meet the surgeon tomorrow. At this time, you will discuss what the next steps will need to be taken."

I had a million questions but remembered that my new friend, the internet, had many of the answers I was looking for. I recall feeling like I had received a big punch to my stomach! My knees buckled and I dropped to the floor. One can never explain the feeling that overtakes us when we find out we have a scary, unpredictable and angry disease like cancer. One feels scared, angry, depressed. I felt like my body had betrayed me.

The next morning, my husband, my mother, and I drove to the surgeon's office. I hadn't slept at all. My head was full of spinning thoughts: I don't want to lose my hair; I don't want to explain this to my kids; I don't want to have cancer; can this all be a bad, bad dream?!

That morning, I realized it was very much not a dream, I walked into his office and right on the table, before he got a word in, was a pamphlet about colon cancer and right hemicolectomy surgery (the removal of 1/2 of my colon).

Dr. Stricheartz looked at me and said, "I assume you know why I called you in here today." I looked at him, confused. "The tumor we found is larger than 95% of people who get carcinoid tumors. Most carcinoids are 1 cm, yours is 2.1 cm and based on its size and statistics of it spreading—upwards of 70% chance of metastasis—we need to go in tomorrow and remove 1/2 your colon."

Another punch to the gut.

The surgery had its complications. I was losing a lot of blood following surgery and they found I was internally hemorrhaging. I had two blood transfusions while a bedside trauma nurse held my hand through the whole thing.

The hemorrhage sealed up on its own.

I spent the next few weeks at home healing. My boys definitely knew something was wrong with Mommy. We tried not to scare them but my fragile state and loss of weight tipped them off. I will never forget my 4-year-old son, Diego, telling my mother during those first few weeks, "Gramma, how old will I be when I get to drive a car?" "You'll be 16, a teenager" pause, "Hmm . . . that's too bad. Mommy will be in heaven when I am a teenager."

Another punch in the gut.

I spent the next several months testing. For someone who spent most of her adult doctor visits in a walk-in clinic, I now had an Internist, an Endocrinologist, a Gastroenterologist, an Oncologist, a Carcinoid Specialist, and a Surgeon. The testing was exhausting! I had a double balloon endoscopy, colonoscopy, endoscopy, swallow camera (that one was actually pretty cool), barium x-rays, regular x-rays. Finally a trip to a Carcinoid Cancer specialist at Cedars Sinai in Los Angeles gave us the answers we were desperately searching for.

After retesting my pathology of my colon, my specialist, Dr. Edward Wolin, informed us of "Small Vessel Lymphatic Invasion." It was stage two; it had left the original location and spread to my lymphatic system.

I would need an octreotide scan, a CT scan, and an MRI, all in one day!

The octreotide image is a nuclear scan. They pump your veins with radioactive dye and you stay completely still for 2 hours. If you move, you start all over again. My nose has never itched so much! I just kept praying and meditating. Once I was done, the radiologist informed me I was the first person in those two hours to not ever press the panic button.. "There was a panic button?!" OMG! I would have most definitely pressed it, had I known.

The octreotide scan showed some "cellular activity" in my abdomen area, perhaps cancer cells, perhaps trauma from the two surgeries; only time will tell. Unfortunately, because carcinoid doesn't respond to chemo and radiation (I get to keep my hair. Yippee!),you need to watch and wait until tumors form and then you do something called debulking. You remove parts or the entire organ it's invaded.

Because of this fact, carcinoid cancer survivors need to be scanned frequently. The good news is it is also known as "cancer in slow motion." The bad news is, who has the patience to "watch and wait" with something as unpredictable as cancer?!

In the past two years, throughout my every-six-month trips to Los Angeles, many things have popped up that need to be checked. I have had a lump in my breast biopsied. It was benign, and more recently a growth in my thyroid that went from .7 cm to 1.7 cm to 2.9 cm in 12 months. As of yesterday's pathology, it is benign yet again.

As with everything I do with my doctors in San Jose, I then need to send it off to my angel Dr. Wolin at Cedars to retest with his special stains and dyes. You see one HUGE lesson I found out: many cancers that are rare may not show up with standard pathology stains. If you have a specific type of cancer, get your scans and pathology done with a specialist. El Camino Hospital sees 1 to 2 carcinoid cases a year, their radiologists maybe perform a handful of octreotide scans a year. Dr. Wolin's team does two to three nuclear scans a day!

Throughout the past two years I have learned a lot about myself, about the people I love, about God, about the power of the human spirit, and about the kindness of strangers, from my carcinoid support group who have become an extension of my family and medical support team to my neighbors who chipped in to bring meals or small gifts for the kids.

Through this process, I needed to take an inventory of my life, my diet, my exercise (or lack of it), my stress levels, even the skincare I use. I know I didn't give myself cancer, but I take ownership of the fact that my tumor was as large as it was, due to the environment I choose to live in. There are toxins in many of our daily products from what I was using on my skin, to my house cleaning products, to the foods I choose to put in my body. I read a book called Ant-Cancer which changed the way I look at food and products. It has helped me regain control over my body, and step up MY role in its health and wellbeing.

In researching the skincare I was using on www.cosmeticsdatabase.com, I discovered that many of the products I was using on myself and my children were dangerous. I knew as a mother, that I needed to become educated on what I was putting on my small boys as well. If our government isn't regulating the 12,000 ingredients in skincare on our shelves, we need to take ownership of it for ourselves and our children.

I do not ever wish to say, cancer is a gift. If cancer is a gift, it's one I would like to return. Rather, what you do with it is your gift to yourself and to others. I choose to be a survivor, to become educated, to take control of my medical care. I get records of every procedure. I study books. I am no longer a victim at an urgent care center. I also now reach out to people who get the stomach-punching news of their own cancer diagnosis. I am now more in the present. The future and past are traps most of us find ourselves in for the bulk of our lives.

I took the passion I had for research and the drive and ambition that fueled my successful career in High Tech Field Sales and I applied it to the research and development of an organic skincare line, and the development of a methodology to rejuvenate skin using eastern medicine and cosmetic acupuncture. To read more about my business visit my site: www.authenticskin.com. It was important to me to give an alternative to the dangerous injectables like Botox*, Juvéderm*, and other toxins which we are now only beginning to see correlations to neurological diseases and other illnesses due to excessive use.

I have merged my passion for health and my passion for beauty and used my fear, my creativity, and my drive to uncover a new way to approach beauty by leveraging the power of the human spirit and searching for authenticity in a plastic, toxin-filled society.

Now, when someone decides to look for toxin-free products on the Cosmeticsdatabase.com, they will find my Authenticskin Remedies products among many of the safe alternatives.

I feel cancer chose me; I have now made the choice to do something with it!

At the time of this book's publication, I am enjoying my baby daughter who just turned two!

Meredith

Time's Spiral and the Journey

Somewhere in elementary school we all sat behind our desks while our teacher drew a straight line across the board and then divided it with two intersecting lines, marking the lineal and logical sequence of time: Past, present and future. This was given as a finite rule of time's reality and we gulped it in, a sweet milky understanding of "what was real".

While we all know that time is really marked by the events in our personal lives (before 9/11 and after 9/11, when I was a kid and now an adult, or before THE CANCER was found and after the cancer was found). We still hold on to the concepts of past, present and future. The exception is if we skip the route, jump the lines and find ourselves in the Spiral's Presence of Present Time, just Now.

This is the metaphysical approach to living life with great gratitude and reverence, because we have let go of any preconceived ideas about what happened in the past and what we wish would occur or what we fear will occur in the future. "Be Here Now" is the mantra (as joyously and creatively as one can be). As a carcinoid journeyer this is my greatest spiritual path on my biggest spiritual journey. It matters little what religious background one had or didn't have or how keyed in you were to appreciating while living in the present, once the doctor comes with the diagnosis of carcinoid whether you are in a hospital room or intimate doctor's office. Time freezes and you enter into the present.

How long you stay there depends on what you do with the journey. For me, I chose to continue on the "present" path, stating my health is in a "healing" condition. Yes, I do make plans that are subject to the present's changes. Yes, I do have future desires, yet I keep them happily engaged in my present's feeling. Yes, above all I am humbled by the kindness in the world, the exquisite pattern of the earth's landscape, the people within it, and I am grateful for being alive and healing day by day.

As a 65 year old artist, I knew how to create something from the blankness of nothing. I knew how to be buoyant in times of changes. I knew how to keep "keeping on".

At the time of the emergency room operation, I had little money in the bank, no permanent home, no savings/investments, no real estate, nor a mate/husband beside me. I did not even have a dependable job or good insurance plan when the cancer specialist doctor entered my hospital room, three days after being entered into the operating room, (operated on for gangrene of the ileum) to bring me fully into the present. This definite carcinoid diagnosis did jump start my life's direction to totally move forward on the spiraling spiritual journey. This journey I call affectionately "Healing in the Now, through Taking Joyous, Creative Baby Steps of Living".

In fact I was in the process of moving to a new rental and buying and selling items on eBay every month (my income), while painting and working on a book of an ancient alphabet. All that stopped for me to begin to take the baby steps of healing.

What I did and do have was family and friends who loved me, an awareness that everything changes and we are capable of great change and improvement (if we don't get into our own "little mindfulness" way). I am grateful to have SOOOO much!

Up to the date of the ER admission, I was in excellent health, looked and felt energetically a good ten to fifteen years younger than my biological age. I did not smoke, drank very little, ate very healthy foods and exercised regularly.

What I did have most of my adult years was a peaceful coexistence with STRESS (from divorces, deaths of family members, and my artistic existence). In fact, just three years previous to my operation, I had extreme stress, although I dealt with it well without medications. Stress did and does take its toll!

I had always had a "tricky" stomach. Sometimes, if I were traveling, I could be constipated for days/weeks if I did not take a laxative. Because of this I ate healthfully and was aware of my body and its changes. Several months before being admitted into the emergency room, I was feeling "odd" in my stomach. I thought it might have been from a hike where I drank the smallest amount of "clear", fast flowing, (melted snow), mountain water. It was a hot Santa Fe, New Mexico summer day and I gave in to my cautious judgment to swallow a small amount from the fast flowing stream. Thinking my stomach problem was a reaction to the stream waters, I visited several doctors, naturopaths, and herbal stores in order to discover what my cramping and diarrhea was about.

I was in the process of taking several remedies after no known cause was found, when one evening I was bent over in excruciating pain. Several hours later a good friend was able took me to the emergency room of a very small local hospital. A CT scan was taken and the operation was ordered.

What the very young surgeon found was a gangrenous ileum and a strangled digestive system and two enlarged cancerous ovaries. He was young, yet skillful and he operated carefully on the digestive system. He then called the hospital's gynecologist to ask whether to remove both or one of the ovaries. The gynecologist, probably not familiar with carcinoid either, said, "just take out one and we'll do a pathology exam on what we find."

The results that came back several days later were clearly mid gut carcinoid with syndrome. After being released from the hospital and staying and resting with a friend for two months while recuperating, I was faced with tremendous changes in diet and lost about 20 pounds.

I still could not manage to control the irregular digestion/ elimination process.

I met with oncologists in Albuquerque, who suggested "trial remedies".

When I read the side effects of these remedies I wasn't ready to jump into Pharma's pool as a "testing" patient. Particularly since there were two "new" drugs being tested, and I had no choice in which one I would be given. I researched one drug and was shown that it caused "suicidal tendencies". When I asked what happens if I become suicidal? The answer given was, "We'll give you drugs to counteract these feelings." It was then that I jumped off the pharma merry-go round, even before the music started.

I began my own alternative health journey. I read everything I could about carcinoid and started searching out and began being treated by several wonderful Native American healers, body work healers, naturopaths, healers of the ancient Japanese acupuncture, like Ho Shin Do, who used live honey bees and their stingers. I was simultaneously going the allopathic route and contacting MD Anderson Cancer center for the possibility of an operation on the remaining ovary, which I felt was impeding my health. I was living in the active and unfolding present. Emotionally, I was a ghost of my former self. I felt removed from any part of my past. I was in a movie, an outsider, an alien to the hustle bustle of the human energy. My previous self? That was then, when I was more carefree and social, more physically active and more in the movement of the general populace of the world (past, present and future).

The first response was from MD Anderson. They said I was "inoperable", so I chose not to go to Houston for further medical discussion of my case (an additional expense, and, as my work was frozen, I was living only on social security's small allowance).

I began looking for a team to operate on the remaining ovarian tumor. Through the internet I found the ACOR group and wrote to the Ochsner Medical Center in Kenner, Louisiana, to begin a healing dialogue. They planned an initial meeting in November, and then surgery would be scheduled in February, if I were to be a surgical candidate. All this was followed by a slew of pre-op additional scans, blood and urine testing and more radioactive tests. This I did not like. However, like many parts of the New Journey, I embraced it. I embraced it after asking myself this leading question, "Is this for my highest and best good?" This question has served me well. It is the present asking me to be fearlessly candid and rely upon my knowledge and trust in the healing journey. It becomes spiritual because the dialogue is inner-directed and one way and is about Life and death, my life and my death!

By late September, I had moved into my own apartment, was working and painting again, resting a lot, and although still extremely thin (I never did regain my lost weight) I could eat a regular meal (reduced in food choices) and even dine out occasionally. I had not yet begun Sandostatin LAR*.

The operation took place in Kenner in February. I traveled there via Denver as there are no direct flights from New Mexico. During a long layover in Denver on my way to the operation I was about to bolt and cancel all plans, when I wrestled with my conscience again: what was my best and highest good? No answer came, as happens when you live in the present. Patience is more than a virtue, it is a way of life. Here I did not have the luxury of time for waiting patiently. Fortunately my traveling companion was my twenty-seven year old, very wise son who was 100% sure that since I was half way there I should go on to Louisiana and the operation.

I must add that my New Mexico oncologist (the third oncologist I have seen) was against having this operation. His thoughts were that it was too invasive and definitely not his choice. The operations would be two operations in less than a year which was too radical for him.

The Kenner surgical team was able to remove 75% of the growth. Nodes were taken off the liver, mesentery wall, and the ovary and gallbladder were removed. The gallbladder was removed because I had finally agreed to begin the Sandostatin LAR® 30 mg. once a month.

After the return home I decided I needed to begin a more active life style and one closer to a larger and more sophisticated medical center. After months of rest I healed slowly and well.

By June I moved to the Space Coast Florida area to stay with my cousin. My brother drove me all the long distance from New Mexico to Florida. We stopped in Louisiana to visit the Kenner surgical team who urged further procedures. These consisted of three chemo-embolizations.

I did not agree to it, as it was not imminent enough for me to do when I asked the question, "Is this to my highest and best good now"?

Upon arriving in Florida, I scheduled an appointment with an oncologist from a large cancer medical center in the area. Three days before the initial meeting, I had a dream of flying as a passenger in a bi-wing, single propeller airplane over the mountains of Colorado. In the dream, we were about to crash into the side of the mountain when the pilot pulled the plane up and over the mountains safely. It surprised me when the next morning I looked at the front page of the local newspaper to see that an air show had taken place in the next town and the cover story photo was a bi-wing plane flying along the coast with condos along the shore below. In fact, it made my dream rush forward in clear detail into my present, from a dreamy and half-forgotten past.

I mentioned this to my cousin at the breakfast table that morning. The real surprise came just three days later at my first Florida oncology visit.

When I arrived at the doctor's inner offices at the cancer center, the only art on the wall was a cartoon portrait of my new oncologist as a pilot in a bi-wing plane. He was waving from the cockpit. There was also an old fashion black and white cut paper silhouette of a bi-wing plane! This to me was more than coincidental!

Upon meeting the oncologist, who said that he flew this type of plane, I felt time was spiraling forward, past to present.

The oncologist was the first doctor to actually say to me that the medical choices were mine. He said that he would be impartial and present my options by tracking my progress. I felt I had entered into another partnership in my healing, one of the many I have been fortunate enough to have.

During the month I have been here I have exercised more than I ever had during the past year and a half, have meditated more, and embraced the present more. At the present time, I am in the Spiral of Healing, staying in the present and on the Healing Spiritual Journey with gratitude, creativity, love, and awareness.

This is a fragment of my story. It has existed with the love and support of family and friends. It exists with a love and innate trust of life, its changes and daily wonders perceived. It exists from a responsible taking of daily baby steps, banishing fears and trusting the process.

As of spring 2012, I am carefully controlling my diet and eating bland foods. Nonetheless, I have had two small bowel obstructions in the past two weeks. My oncologist recently told me "There is nothing else I can do for you". I was shocked and asked about clinical trials. I am intending to pursue PRRT in Europe.

As my bowel obstructions continued, I had the choice of a peg tube into my stomach for feedings and or TPN (total parenteral nutrition). I chose TPN and am now living with my brother. I have my own room but am getting weaker and losing weight. I think I have another bowel obstruction. My friend Maria G. from San Francisco and my friend Caren from Santa Fe call me on a daily basis. I am beginning to become afraid but, yet, I embrace what is.

I am continuing to lose weight and as I can't eat anything my mouth, I took a chance one day, as I am so hungry. I ate a quesadilla and almost immediately developed severe abdominal pain and nausea. I told Maria that the quesadilla was probably going to hurt me, but it tasted so good. She never judged my choice.

Sadly, our Meredith, living with her brother in Atlanta, passed away on July 14th, 2012

> *The fear of death follows from the fear of life.*
> *A man who lives fully is prepared to die at any time.*
> —Mark Twain

Jennifer

Diagnosed: Feb/March 2010
Type: Midgut carcinoid cancer
Stage: 4 (carcinoid syndrome and suspected carcinoid heart disease)
Age: 40

I went to the doctor in December 2009 thinking I either had gall stones or ulcers due to strong upper abdominal pain. It felt like I was being punched in the stomach. By the end of February 2010, we found and biopsied the primary carcinoid tumor in my small intestine (ileum). At that point, I had also lost my appetite and felt nauseous most of the time. I had my first OctreoScan™ in March, which showed hot spots on my liver too. In April, I had surgery to remove six inches of my small intestine, ascending colon and half of my transverse colon. They took out sixteen lymph nodes—nine had been invaded by cancer. And they took out the two tumors on my liver.

As my oncologist and I looked back on my history, in 2004 I started seeing a GI doctor for upper abdominal pain and diarrhea. That same year I started seeing a cardiologist due to a tachycardia arrhythmia and fainting due to drops in blood pressure (along with flushing). In 2008, I developed thickened valves (all 4 valves) in my heart, which remain unchanged to date.

We were hoping that the surgery would get rid of my stomach pain and I'd magically feel better. That was not the case. By the end of May 2010, I was rushed to the ER in the most excruciating upper abdominal pain I've had yet. The ER docs had no idea what the cause was. I continue to have these pain attacks, the cause of which no one can find. My gallbladder went bad in June 2011. I had a PowerPort˙ put in during that surgery. It has helped out so much! But the removal of my gallbladder did not "cure" the pain attacks.

I have spent a minimum of 3 days in the hospital once a month since January of 2012. The longest time I have spent in the hospital was 2 weeks. These may not be all related to carcinoid, but I have gone into carcinoid crisis.

By September 2011, the OctreoScan™ showed "significant uptake" (mets) in my upper middle chest area. We're still waiting on labs to come back. I also have to have my heart re-evaluated to see if there is any progression of the valve thickening. I'm on Sandostatin LAR˙ injections every twenty days at 30 mg., rescue shots of octreotide, Creon˙ (pancreatic enzymes), Metformin (for pre-diabetics to try to help prevent diabetes), and a medication for my heart, which tends to bottom out my blood pressure. I have low blood pressure readings as it is. I've also have migraines and mood swings associated with carcinoid cancer.

I try to take everything day by day. I went on long-term disability from work in August of 2010. Between the fatigue, attacks of abdominal pain (can't function while on pain meds), continued diarrhea, and tons of doctor appointments, scans, and tests, there's not enough time to work full time at this point. I don't have anywhere near the energy I used to have. On a good day I have maybe a three hour window. I'm grateful every day that I'm in my home and with my family and not "living" in the hospital. I've have even been able to take a few trips with them.

I am currently awaiting a diagnosis for multiple enlarged lymph nodes that have increased in size and number since March of 2012. I have been told that lymphoma or another disease may account for the enlarged nodes. I do not have a diagnosis at this time but have been referred to Mayo clinic for further studies. I am having fevers, sweats that are drenching, abdominal pain, occasional diarrhea and profound fatigue. When I have the sweats, which occur sporadically, I also have chills, shortness of breath, chest pain and total body itching without evidence of rashes.

I am hopeful that the doctors at Mayo find out what is going on with me, as my symptoms have increased and I am SO tired of no one being able to tell me what is going on or knowing how to treat me. These new issues are basically destroying my life. I await my appointment at the Mayo Clinic.

"Life is about the journey, not the destination."

"Don't take life too seriously—no one gets out alive."

Bill Evans

"C" is for Carcinoid—My Carcinoid Story

June 2003

My experience with carcinoid cancer began in January 1995, although I did not know it at the time. I had a heart attack followed by a couple of small strokes. The medications prescribed by my primary physician masked symptoms we now recognize are related to carcinoid syndrome. The doctor expressed the opinion that my flushing and diarrhea were related to undesired but not unexpected effects of the medications I was on.

During the next seven and half years I voiced my concerns over the ever increasing symptoms to both my primary care physician and the heart doctor. Each time I was pronounced as being in extremely good shape . . . for a man of my age and medical history.

By March 2002, the diarrhea had advanced to the point that it was socially embarrassing. This prompted an "early retirement" as I could not leave my home office very often. Going to meals with business associates and friends had been dwindling due to the embarrassing flushing events when my neck, face and head became extremely red and always created comments at the table.

By now I was becoming weak, listless and apathetic. I had started a consulting business to work out of my home office during hours I wanted and doing the kind of work I wanted to do. Even with that freedom, I just didn't feel like doing anything and the symptoms got worse.

In May I knew something was terribly wrong. After all this time, my doctors could not or would not even look into the possibility of something else causing my problems. So I contacted the Sansum Clinic in Santa Barbara, California, and made an appointment for a complete examination. During the initial interview the physician narrowed down my problem to one of three possibilities and ordered tests to isolate the cause of my distress.

The tests indicated it was the worst possible cause, carcinoid cancer. I still recall the shock of hearing the word "cancer" for the first time, as it related to my condition. We had been discussing the possibility of a tumor but this was the first time it was suggested it was other than benign.

They determined the "primary location" was in the mid-gut and recommended surgery. We took that under advisement as my family and I returned to our home to consider all the options. During the next several days the pain grew worse each time I would eat and create "movement" in the intestines. The main cancer mass and tumor was located at the point where the small intestine meets the colon and it failed to show on all tests with the exception of a CT scan. This scan also showed that the liver was fully involved with over 20 tumors.

We accepted the doctor's recommendation for surgery and in late August 2002 a considerable amount of my internal parts were removed. A biopsy of these parts revealed carcinoid cancer was involved in each one. The doctors stated the tumors in the liver were too advanced for surgical procedures. For the first time we learned that this was incurable and inoperable.

The only good news was that it was a "slow growing" cancer. I asked what that meant. Did that mean I got to live longer with the problem, or take longer to die than those with "fast growing" cancer? Why can't the liver be operated on? Why isn't it curable? I also asked many more questions that all support the denial portion of my journey. This passed quickly but it was still a shock.

I began a regimen of Sub-Q Sandostatin* injections for carcinoid syndrome in November 2002 and Testosterone for physical weakness in February 2003. It has been reported that in time the Sandostatin* may lose some of its effectiveness. In the beginning to intermediate stages this can sometimes be estimated, but in advanced cases such as mine, well, no one knows. We all take it one day at a time. After a few months we switched to monthly Sandostatin LAR* injections.

A very old report stated that, statistically, life expectancy from the onset of symptoms was around 7.42 years. Just about the same amount of time the doctors ignored my symptoms and complaints. It has now been over 17 years since the symptoms began and although my case is in an advanced stage, I am still here and able to function. OK, not like before, but then I am not confined to 30 paces from my toilet. I eat a lot of things I simply could not before the surgery and medications, and that is a big improvement.

I have avoided documenting the details and statistics of my journey with carcinoid cancer since every case seems to be as unique as the individual. What we are all interested in is what will happen next. Will there be pain? How long do I have? No one is comfortable discussing these issues, but yet that is what we all want to know.

Here is the answer, but I warn you: it is not very satisfying. It differs for each person. Your journey is just that, your journey. The end of your life is as unique as how you lived it. Not everyone lives exactly the same or passes the same. How this will end for others is not necessarily how it will end for you.

When I was born, 65 was the life expectancy for most children in the United States. Therefore, that number has had a special meaning for me throughout my life. My Dad died at age 55, just before his 56th birthday and I wondered if I would make it to my "allotted" time. God has been good and I indeed did make it to 65 and beyond.

It may be important to point out that maintaining a positive attitude is very helpful. There is always hope. Hope for a cure, a significant delay, a reversal, anything that will help you feel better. Yet we all know that someday this life's journey will come to a close. Don't let the illness defeat you. It is a major problem but your whole life is not the cancer. It is just one of the many things you have to deal with, and you have dealt with a lot of other issues in your life. So keep on keeping on.

Believing that every life story should have a moral, or at least a purpose, here is my encouragement to anyone reading this and trying to learn more about carcinoid cancer.

Take responsibility for your own body! Doctors are very much like any other professionals. They can advise, but it is YOU that must decide! They are busy doing a fantastic job for the most part, and society is, and should be, indebted to those in this profession. But, they are not perfect, and, given their case loads, insurance companies, government regulations, etc. they do a wonderful job. Only YOU know your body and how you feel. Don't accept fast answers if it just doesn't seem right. Get another opinion.

Don't wait too long! If I had acted upon my condition a few years before I did, I might have a good chance of extending my life expectancy, not to mention the quality of life (and kept my innards).

Don't let the condition dominate your entire life. As long as you are alive, live!

Do not accept defeat. Only you can let yourself be defeated.

When I learned about my condition, I wrote the item below and during these past few years my opinion has not wavered. If you find some comfort from this, then please use it to your best advantage.

May God continue to bless and keep you and yours.

Bill

Death has not conquered!

I have been released! Released from a body that was in decay, growing weaker, and would have given out at some point in the future anyway. I have been restored! I am in a new body as promised by my Lord Jesus Christ.

I am reconciled with my Lord for eternity.

I am remembered by so many loving and caring friends and family and I will continue to live in their hearts.

I am grateful to my God for the privilege of having a wonderful life.

I thank my God for the opportunity to learn and grow the way He wanted.

I had many failures but only one victory was necessary and He provided that!

I don't want to start a list of those I have loved and who love me, but of course the one person that cannot be ignored is Margie, my very best friend and companion for life. We took a vow that we have lived every day. As a result, we truly became one as God has so ordered in His Word. All of His blessings were bestowed upon us. No one has ever had it better than we did.

My life was one of complete contentment. God filled every need. My wife and I loved each other completely. So I ask, "How could death possibly conquer?" Once again, God has the final victory. To Him I give my life. A poor offering indeed, but it is what He asked for.

(The above was written when I was given my "death sentence". My status has changed, the thoughts have not. This is and will be valid in the future.)

In 2004 and 2005, Bill participated in a clinical trial of a new drug designed for carcinoid cancer and allowed highly skilled surgeons to remove 75% of his liver, reducing the number of tumors to four. A recent MRI now shows eleven tumors in the liver and several in the pelvic area. In April 2008 Bill agreed to participate in another clinical trial of a new drug coded RAD001 (now marketed as Afinitor'). Results are highly favorable.

Bill spends much of his time helping others to learn about carcinoid and cope with the impact of the disease. He welcomes inquiries for data: billmargie@comcast.net

Sadly, Bill passed away on October 31, 2012.

> *"And God will wipe away every tear from their eyes; there shall be no more death, nor sorrow, nor crying. There shall be no more pain, for the former things have passed away."*
> —*Revelation 21:4*

Linda

It's important to begin with some history. I had symptoms of irritable bowel syndrome since my mid 40's. This is important to remember as it is part of the history for many people diagnosed with carcinoid. Of course, I believed my doctor but never received any real fix for my condition. I had off-and-on diarrhea, but never anything that interfered with my life. I also had, on occasion, bloated constipation, and I just dealt with it.

Fast forward:

Here I am, an athletic woman in her mid 50's, independent, and moving to Belize to retire from the taxes and hurry-up life of the United States. I have two wonderful daughters, who are now married and on their own life journeys. I figured it was now my time to explore a little and give that free spirit artist inside me a run for her money. I sold my condo on the central coast of California beach, my business, and the equipment. I exchanged it all for the freedom to live the island life and paint the tropics. Ah, Paradise! The first two years were lovely. I was diving, sailing, losing weight (had diarrhea occasionally), and felt on top of the world. I was meeting new people from all over the world and had myself a nice little gallery on the beach. My art was selling well.

Then I began feeling tired, a lot tired. I figured it was from all the work and acclimating to the tropics and my new, busy, lifestyle. Most the time I felt great, but in hindsight, the symptoms were slowly creeping up on me, kind of when one gets fat slowly and doesn't really notice until it is there big time.

About the third year of living in Belize, I began having weird bouts of diarrhea, feeling very fatigued and having weird hot flashes that were worse than my menopause. Living in the tropics with the heat and humidity, I questioned my feelings. Finally I went to some local doctors who, of course, equated my symptoms to menopause. The last doctor I decided to try was a well-respected female doctor from Cuba. I thought maybe she would be a better choice and would not excuse my symptoms as "menopausal". The hot flash symptom became very strange: a feeling that my face was growing outward and a pulse inside my mouth that included my gums. I'd experience a huge pressure surge that would subside after several seconds. I also began having horrible diarrhea. The doctor ran some tests for a parasite and found I did have one. I took the medicines for the parasite and was successful with a full recovery. The diarrhea and weird flushes continued, however. Blood tests and several other exams were done with nothing rearing its ugly head.

She sent me to the city to a cardiologist because I told her about the heart palpitations I would feel during this weird rush. My heart tests all came out fine, including a 24 hour monitor. My heart skipped beats once in a while, but nothing to worry about. Another dead end. The doctor wanted to do a colonoscopy, but I thought I would look into things once I got back to the U.S. I found myself having times of confusion or inability to multitask. I knew something else was going on. I had thoughts that the parasite had entered my brain.

Because of other matters, I chose to return to the U.S.A. I had an urgent feeling that I must get home. Back in California by December 2010, my daughter said that I was acting differently. I didn't know what she meant. Every time I would raise my heartbeat at the gym, I would get those horrible hot flashes that would take my breath away and my heart pounded almost uncontrollably. I was engaged and married on Valentine's Day 2011. By June of 2011, my husband encouraged me to see our primary doctor as he was seeing rapid changes in my skin and overall appearance. I had been complaining how tired I was all the time. We both thought that maybe the parasite I got in the tropics was ravishing my body. My doctor immediately sent me for a CT scan. Three hours later I got a call from him, "Mrs. B. I am sending you to an oncologist. You have three tumors!"

Turns out my oncologist was familiar with carcinoid cancer and suspected what was wrong. The first thing out of his mouth was, "Linda, do you get really horrible hot flashes?" I immediately began to cry in fear and in joy that finally someone was listening to me.

I have had carcinoid for approximately eight to ten years. Now the cancer has followed its recognized course and metastasized to my liver. My oncologist sent me to a southern California hospital for surgery. They addressed a second type of cancer on my left kidney by laparoscope, and removed the ileum of my small intestine, a portion of my large bowel (my primary tumor), and appendix. The surgeon neglected to follow orders and remove my gall bladder in preparation for receiving Sandostatin˚.

Following surgery, my surgeon pulled my husband aside in the waiting room and told him that if he had known prior to surgery, he wouldn't have bothered operating since my abdomen was scattered with rice like appearing tumors. He then told my husband, "she has six weeks to live. Take her home and make her comfortable." So much for knowledgeable surgeons!

Please, question every doctor and have tests done outside the box. I wished I had.

Somebody should tell us,
right at the start of our lives, that we are dying.
Then we might live life to the limit,
every minute of every day.
Do it! I say.
Whatever you want to do, do it now!
There are only so many tomorrows.
—Pope Paul VI, 1897-1978

Haydee

I am a 70 year old woman (never thought I would get this far) and looking back have probably had carcinoid (whoa! I am counting with my fingers) over thirty years. I keep a log of everything, because every time I have to see a doctor they ask me for my "curriculum" as I call it. In 1981, 1983, and 1992 I had atypical pneumonia. All through those years, and before, I suffered from what doctors told me was a spastic intestine. Since I often was under much stress, I took their word for it. At that time I was living in Tegucigalpa, Honduras with my husband and raising three boys. I lived there from 1996 to 2002. Honduras was not a very "modern" country and due to its proximity to the U.S we traveled there for more serious medical problems.

In 1994 I had a collapsed lung and an x-ray finally showed an undefined mass in my left lung. For years I had been treated for asthma because I coughed a lot. I inhaled medication, and at the end, often had to sleep sitting up, but nothing calmed this cough which at times was quite bad. I had several lung X-rays. I even traveled to Miami to see a lung specialist. I had a biopsy with inconclusive results and surgery was planned. In August 1994, I had a bronchial carcinoid tumor removed as well as the left lower lobe of my lung. I was told by the surgeon that all was clear and that I would no longer have any

153

problems, because this was a benign tumor. After the removal of the tumor my intestinal cramps and occasional diarrhea slowly stopped, my digestion improved and I stopped coughing.

In July 1997, I had very painful cramps and stool tests for amoeba were done (I lived in a country where we had many parasites) as well as a 24-hour urine test for carcinoid. My level for the urine tests had always been very low. Several months later I had such strong cramps that I went to the emergency room but the wait was so long, (and I had taken pain medication) that I finally left without being seen by a doctor. I was not bleeding to death, so they just made me wait! At that time I was spending much of my time in Miami, so I took advantage and went to see a very good family doctor who immediately ordered an ultrasound of my abdomen. She thought I might have gall or kidney stones. Radiology suggested a CT scan because they saw something in my liver. This showed metastatic disease or a liver cyst. Both proved to be true later on.

In the meantime I was back home in Honduras, and we decided to go to MD Anderson in the spring of 1998. They did a series of tests, including a liver biopsy, which confirmed carcinoid mets. I was told to come back in three months, that this was a slow-developing disease, that I would probably live a long time and die of something else. I returned in July 1998 to go through the same and be told to come back in another three months. Of course I could not be traveling every three months to be told the same thing and sit in the hospital for a day or two. In the meantime my sons started doing research and pushing me to do the same and read what they had found on carcinoid tumors. Slowly it dawned on my husband and me that we had to take this disease in hand and be more pro-active.

Through the support group and S. Anderson, I got in contact with Dr. Warner in New York and started seeing him in May of 1999. One of our sons was already living in New York and was a great support. Dr. Warner ordered an OctreoScan™ which showed multiple carcinoid tumors in the liver. In June, I had liver tumor resection and cryo-ablation at Mt. Sinai Hospital in N.Y. Dr. Shafir was the surgeon and he also performed gall bladder resection because I was going to be put on Sandostatin* three times a day. After surgery, I started Sandostatin LAR* at 30 mg. per month. Dr. Shafir could not remove all of the tumors, however. In August 1999 I also started interferon alpha three times a week. I had to stop it in March, 2000, because I was completely fuzzy in my head, had trouble forming sentences and completing my thoughts. I walked around like an old woman, and on top of it all, it did not reduce my tumors.

In April 2000 I began a series of three arterial chemo-embolizations at Mr. Sinai Hospital, N.Y. I completed them in September. Dr. Warner supervised all the treatments and I was very glad to have chosen him as my doctor. I returned to Honduras and continued seeing Dr. Wang in Miami for my checkups, scans and lab tests. I also continued to visit Dr. Warner once a year.

In 2002 we sold our home in Honduras and moved to Buenos Aires were my mother lived. We sold our businesses. Two of our sons lived in Brooklyn and one in São Paulo, Brazil we wanted to live in a more civilized country and care for my mother. We still traveled often to Miami and New York. A scan I had in Miami in the fall of 2004 indicated a tumor in my right humerus. I had surgery in Buenos Aires in May 2006 to remove part of my right humerus and the insertion of titanium prosthesis. Biopsy confirmed carcinoid tumor. Unfortunately the surgery was not a complete success because I have limited use of my arm, but have learned to manage it well and can do practically everything except reach up. Fortunately, I am ambidextrous.

In April 2006, my six-month CT showed a growth in my right kidney and a needle biopsy came back as carcinoid. I went back to New York to see Dr. Warner. He suggested radio-frequency ablation (RFA) and I went to see his interventional radiologist. I asked for advice from my nephew who is a liver transplant surgeon. He told me that this kind of treatment was risky because it could burn more than what was necessary. Therefore, Dr. Warner sent me to a kidney surgeon and I had surgery in May. In August 2006 I started six cycles of chemotherapy with Xeloda* and Temodar.* This treatment was completed in January 2007.

Since then, apparently, I have had no new tumors. My husband injects me with Sandostatin LAR* 30 mg. every 28 days, and I get CT scans of my lungs, abdomen and pelvis every 6 months. I have found two doctors here in Argentina who have carcinoid patients and they attend conferences in Europe on NETs. I get annual heart checkups at a cancer institute where they record the heart ultrasounds of carcinoid patients for comparative and statistical studies. Recently it became possible to have Chromogranin A blood tests done at a public hospital. My numbers have remained very low, and I no longer have the 24-hour urine 5-HIAA test done. I imagine they are no longer used for these tumors, although when I first contacted Dr. Warner it was because my urine index had been very low and then it doubled in value.

I still take the vitamins Dr. Warner prescribed from the onset: Niacin, a multivitamin, Fish Oil, and now I also take Lipitor for my cholesterol and even if I resist, I will probably have to take something for my sugar level which is a bit high.

I wish to add that I have a wonderful family who is always there to support and help me. My husband had just retired when I had liver surgery and he took excellent care of me, doing all the household chores and shopping. After that surgery, I slept practically for a whole month.

Do keep safe and healthy.

> *"I can be changed by what happens to me.*
> *But I refuse to be reduced by it."*
> —*Maya Angelou*

S. L. Anderson

Trials and Tribulations of "Sunny Susan"

I am a survivor of a neuroendocrine cancer called carcinoid. I was diagnosed in May of 1995. I am also a breast cancer survivor and type II diabetic. Fortunately for those of us with carcinoid, it is a slow growing cancer or the majority of us would have died before the diagnosis was made. I am thankful that I have always been an optimist, seeing the glass as half full versus half empty. This has empowered me to become an advocate for carcinoid cancer awareness, which includes self-help support groups for patients and their families as well as having a website devoted to carcinoid cancer. You can visit at www.carcinoidinfo.info which I started in April of 1997. This website was the first informative website put up by a carcinoid patient and a volunteer labor of love on my part. The website includes names of carcinoid specialists, updates in the field, local carcinoid support groups, humor, books, bluegrass, and my travel adventures.

My quest for a diagnosis began in 1987. After years of searching for the cause of upper and lower abdominal pain, a small bowel enteroclysis was carried out. It revealed the need for surgery due to an obstruction. During surgery, May 10, 1995, 85 cm of intestine, 6 lymph nodes from my small bowel (mid ileum) were removed. Metastasis was found in my liver. I finally had a diagnosis—CARCINOID CANCER. I remained in the hospital for ten days, and was very happy to finally have a diagnosis. Not knowing what was wrong with me, plus the pain and weight loss, was terrible! It was very hard on me since I am a researcher, and a "take charge type" and a very active, controlling person. I am a type A personality and an ESTJ on the Myers-Briggs personality indicator. I finally had a diagnosis so I was finally able to start researching this cancer called carcinoid.

The previous six months up until May 1995, I had lived on ice cream, milk shakes and vomited when I tried to eat anything else. I was in severe, constant pain, and lost 62 pounds. I was told I was "paranoid" after gall-bladder surgery: this pain was all in my head. I had bright red "flushing" of the face, neck, chest and arms, which doctors ignored when my husband and I would mention this symptom. As I learned, I would not be flushing without metastasis to my liver.

Over the years I consulted with several doctors, admitted to the hospital many times for partial bowel blockages. I underwent multiple tests in search for answers. Testing included: upper and lower GI's, ultrasound of liver, pancreas and abdomen, sigmoidoscopy, colonoscopy, barium enema with air, CTs of chest, abdomen, pelvis, gastrointestinal endoscopy, stomach lining biopsy, liver biopsy, chest x-rays, mammograms, hydrogen breath test, gall bladder surgery, small bowel enteroclysis, and many blood tests. I NEVER had testing that would have shown the presence of a neuroendocrine tumor (Chromogranin-A, Serotonin, etc.).

Since then I have had several bone density scans, a bone marrow biopsy, nuclear OctreoScans™, heart echocardiograms, heart stress tests, MRIs and various other studies. During the final six months before diagnosis, I had very difficult decisions to make. Due to my health status, I had to resign from six organizations and/or boards I served on and missed the meetings of two book discussion groups.

There are two major problems for those of us dealing with carcinoid cancer. First of all, getting a correct diagnosis of carcinoid, or any of the neuroendocrine cancers, is difficult. Most doctors only see one or two cases in their years of practice and thus do not think to test for these cancers. Secondly, finding a local oncologist who is secure and forward thinking enough to consult one of the few world carcinoid "experts" can be problematic.

It has been said that carcinoid is the "look good cancer." Most of us look healthy and others cannot tell that we have a terminal disease. Carcinoid is one of the more costly cancers to treat because many people live with it for years or decades, thus enduring long-term treatment costs.

My search on the internet began in May 1995. My quest for information yielded mostly outdated information and I refused to accept what I read. I read that with a diagnosis of carcinoid I had only from two to five years to live. I saw four doctors in Arizona. All were "wait and see—do nothing" doctors. I had the same "complaints"—pain in various places, diarrhea, constant and severe fatigue, as well as weakness. I was told many times that carcinoid is a "chronic illness" and to "learn to live with it". No, I could not accept that passive role!

My search for the cause of my stomach and abdominal pain began in 1987 and ended in 1998 when I consulted, in person, with one of the world's leading experts on carcinoid. He is Dr. Richard R. P. Warner from New York City. He is Medical Director of the Carcinoid Cancer Foundation, Inc., chartered in 1968. (www.carcinoid.org). He turned my life around! I am fortunate to have this incredible medical team: Dr. Warner, Dr. Jack Cavalcant, Dr. Sandra Levitt and Dr. Matthew Borst. The latter three are in my home town in Arizona.

After my diagnosis, I felt a very strong desire to assist others in their search for information and in starting local self-help support groups. Since I have always reached out to assist others, it was only normal for me to share with others the information I had found through research. I have never been bored a day in my life and never have enough hours in the day or days in the week. I now maintain 77 mailing-lists in my computer address book of people who either have carcinoid or an interest in the disease. I send information to all of my mailing-lists when new research papers by carcinoid expert doctors or notices about upcoming conferences are available. I also have additional mailing lists for books, humor, good things to think about, politics and Bluegrass music.

In April 1997, I put up my web site carcinoidinfo.info. This is a volunteer labor of love on my part and all cost is happily covered by my husband and me. I provide information for medical / drug databases, information from leading carcinoid doctors on how to treat and monitor carcinoid, local carcinoid support groups, humor, books, Bluegrass music, religion, travel, political issues, Arizona information, cowboy poetry, genealogy, and much more that may assist a person in leading a full and active life while LIVING with carcinoid. There are links to information I wish had been on when I started my research. I am happy to assist others in their quest for information and understanding, not only from my web site, but from the many links available. When this page was fourteen years old in April 2011, there had been 311,410 "visits" to it. I plan to maintain this site for at least another decade.

I believe many of us can lead a full and active life while LIVING with cancer, and/or other chronic conditions. My Type A personality combined with my natural born optimism helps.

I have made many "friends without faces" from around the world via the internet and am fortunate to have met many of these on-line friends at conferences and other places over the years. I appreciate each and every one of these interesting and courageous people I know personally or am in contact with. They have enriched my life and continue to do so!

From my experience, conferences are important in that we can get to meet and learn new information from carcinoid specialists and meet people from all over the world. We get to network with old and new friends, and learn that we are not alone in battling our cancer.

I have attended seven conferences and served on the board of California Carcinoid Fighters Seminar in Santa Ana, California in 2003. In Berlin, Germany I spoke about my web site and forming local support groups. I was on a panel of long-time survivors (I prefer to say "winners") at the September 2005 conference in Philadelphia,

PA. I was also at the Portland, Oregon National conference in 2006 as a speaker. My husband Howard spoke on his "caregiver experience".

I believe anyone with a diagnosis of carcinoid cancer, or ANY kind of cancer needs to be pro-active and assertive. We may be assertive without being disagreeable. The key is practicing "The Golden Rule" by being pleasant, and nice to everyone at all times. At the same time, we must be persistent and clear in requesting what we want done. We are entitled to all of our medical reports, knowledge about treatment expectations and answers relevant to our cancer.

All doctors and their staff are much like you and me. They deal with stress and heavy work-loads. I advise you to be polite, kind and considerate with them. We want and need our care givers to be our allies and not dread seeing our name on the appointment sheet!

Dr. Warner started me on Sandostatin˙ (octreotide acetate) in early 1998, eventually switching me to Sandostatin LAR˙ (long acting release). In 1999 he added interferon Alfa 2-b. I am currently on Peg Intron-A. This joint treatment, along with my second very extensive surgery in October 1999, has kept me stable. I continue to have my routine tests related to carcinoid cancer as well as healthcare maintenance issues addressed.

When a doctor ignores our questions or appears to not show interest in the latest research regarding our cancer, or does not consult with medical experts and may even tell patients "learn to live with it", then it is time to find a different physician. We need a provider who is caring, treats his patients as people versus numbers and is not ego attached.

The way I have chosen to manage my carcinoid is to be pro-active, and it may not be the plan for everyone. We all must find our own way in choosing how we want to be treated. There is no right or wrong way, only different ways. The plan I have shared with you works for me. It may not be the path you choose. Those who research and learn about their disease do much better than those who want the doctor and family to make all of the decisions for them.

I organized my first book discussion group in February 1962 (The Study Guild in Osceola, MO), and am a voracious reader. I organized two book groups when we moved to Arizona in 1983. I maintain the records of these groups. At these monthly meeting I feel as though I am "recharging my batteries", as the participants have lived all over the world and I enjoy learning new things.

We've hosted weekly traditional acoustic Bluegrass music jam sessions in our home in Arizona for 25 years and 6 years before that in Virginia. In 2009, we moved the jam sessions to once a month. I send e-mail to a wide audience with information on upcoming Bluegrass music festivals and events.

My husband, Howard and I are parents of three adult children (one in Arkansas, one in Florida and one in Arizona). We have seven grandchildren. We both had earlier marriages and feel our happy lives really began with our marriage in December 1970. We have many interests we enjoy: art, concerts, theater, music, sunsets, animals, nature, politics, astronomy, camping, travel, and my genealogical research. We accomplished my life-long dream of driving the Al-Can Highway to and from Alaska in 2007, a three and a half month motor home trip.

I've been blessed with being able to travel extensively and enjoy life with my husband Howard. We have visited or cruised to multiple countries, all 50 states in America, and have seen some incredible parts of this earth. Please see my "Travel" section on my website for the latest photographs at www.carcinoidinfo.info. Travel is our way of celebrating life and we enjoy it so much.

We "camp" (in a small motor home) here in Arizona, often taking my husband's 10" telescope so he can take deep space photographs seen at www.astroshow.com. We also "camp" at Bluegrass Festivals and Bluegrass music campouts. We enjoy travel and the outdoors, in addition to art, music, history, science, books and new technology. We both like to constantly learn new things.

Every person has to choose his or her passion. Ours is a demonstration of what keeps us vital and thriving. I will repeat that I believe in "The Golden Rule" and try to practice it in all I do.

There have never been enough hours in the day for me. I have no way of knowing how long I will have this level of GOOD quality of life (pain-free and energetic). My goal is to make the most of each day, count my blessing, have some good "belly laughs", read newspapers, magazines and books, review positive poems, quotes and good things to think about, and above all, assist others.

I fully expect to die of "old age" and not "carcinoid" (I turned 75 in December 2012). I remain optimistic about my future, and know I am richly blessed. Life IS good. As my wonderful husband Howard says, "Each day is a gift"!

Last year, I was awarded the Monica Warner award for self-advocacy, and, I must say, I was both surprised and elated to receive it. My goal is to help others, and to be commended this way is an honor!

Because I can no longer ignore death,
I pay more attention to life.

—Treya Wilber

"Humankind has not woven the web of life. We are but
one thread within it. Whatever we do to the web, we do to
ourselves. All things are bound together. All things connect."

—Chief Seattle

S.A.C.

13 Ways Tough!

I started having what I call feminine problems years ago: painful menstrual cycles that left me curled up in a fetal position, crying myself to sleep. I experienced abdominal pain before and during bowel movements. I went to doctor after doctor, getting told there was nothing wrong with me. I came to believe this to be normal. Every couple of months I would get so tired that I would sleep for two days straight. I decided it was because I stayed so busy and just needed the extra rest. At the time, I took care of an elderly couple. I played the role of housekeeper, gardener, driver and companion. We would schedule and sometimes re-schedule events around my 'sick' days.

Towards the end of 2009, my sick days were becoming more frequent. I couldn't function the same as I had been, so I decided to go to the emergency room at W.O. Moss Regional Hospital. It was then I was told I had cysts on my ovaries. I met with my team of four ob-gyn doctors that I would come to respect and even love.

I was in so much pain that when the doctor suggested surgery to stop the pain, I agreed. Surgery was scheduled for October 29, 2009. I got up around 4:00 a.m. and got ready to head to the hospital. While I was lying in bed, the surgeon came in to talk to me and asked if I had any kids and I told him no. He asked if I wanted kids and I told him yes. Surgery was cancelled. I didn't know I was about to have a hysterectomy. I'm grateful he came to talk to me before. All I heard was "make the pain go away," and I was on board, not even knowing what I was agreeing to. On October 31st I had laparoscopic surgery to remove the cysts. All went well and I was released the next day.

Five days later, I was right back in the emergency room in excruciating pain. I was rushed back into surgery, where, in an effort to preserve my fertility, only my right tube and ovary were removed. It was said that a cyst had erupted in my right fallopian tube but that everything was alright. I disagreed! I was now hurting all the time and felt like I was having my cycle every day of the month. I could no longer function like a normal person (whatever normal was!). During a visit with one of my gynecologists, he was going to do a biopsy on my uterus but when I started crying, he stopped. He said he didn't want to put me in any more pain and suggested I have the hysterectomy after all. This time I knew what I was agreeing to. Because of the waiting list at Moss, surgery wasn't scheduled till the following year.

I decided to do some research, since I had a few months to prepare myself for what was about to happen. I went to the library and started reading books on menopause and it kind of freaked me out! Do women really go through this—hot flashes, mood swings, needing to take hormones; different kinds of hormones? I read all I could and wasn't feeling any better about it, but, since it was going to happen eventually anyways, I decided to take it like a woman and not a wuss! I asked for advice from other women who were in their change. I became confident that I could do this gracefully.

About two weeks before my hysterectomy, I found myself in the emergency room yet again. I had what was called an abscess in my vagina. The emergency room doctor drained it, but nobody really knew what it was or why it was there. I was admitted to the hospital where the abscess was surgically removed, and I was released the next day. Two weeks later, I was in the holding room talking about it, and the gynecologist said that in all his years, he's never heard of that happening, but he'd take a look at my chart and see if there was anything there during surgery.

I woke up, happy to have a morphine drip. It was finally over. After healing, there would be no more pain. No more crying myself to sleep. No more curling up in a ball and rocking. I was fixed! After a few days, I thought I'd be released but I wasn't. Dr. Darby said they wanted to run more tests and keep me a little longer because of the abscess that was removed. I was quarantined and a doctor from the Center for Disease Control (CDC) came to examine me. Nobody could figure me out. Tests were coming back normal. The abscess was not in anyone's book. Nothing about it made sense.

Surgery went well, however, my bowels were stuck together (whatever that meant), so that had to be fixed (meaning cut apart). Normally after a hysterectomy, patients stay in the hospital a few days, go home and come back to have the staples removed. Not me. I was kept in the hospital for two more weeks until they took out my staples. I was told I would have drainage but I didn't. I went to a crab boil at my sister's house, and I felt warm and wet on my belly. Fluid was pouring out of my incision. Back to the emergency room I went. When I stood up, a stream of yellowish liquid sprayed two feet in front of me. My incision was cleaned and packed

By now it's April 2010, and when I went back to the doctor for a checkup, they treated me weird. The nurse came and got me out of the waiting room instead of calling my name over a loud speaker. I followed her up and down the hall looking for an empty room. Finally we found one that had two chairs in it, so we went in and sat down. The nurse acted kind of strange: stumbling over her words so I told her, "Hey . . . I'm a big girl, just say what's on your mind."

Her next words changed my life forever, "You have cancer." I was stunned. My mind couldn't understand. I started crying. Everyone I knew with cancer was dead! I'm too young to die. I'm 37. I haven't lived yet. In just a few minutes, a million thoughts went through my head. I sucked it up, dried my eyes and asked the nurse, "What do we do now?" She told me they wanted to send me to Shreveport, four hours away, to find out what kind of cancer I had. Apparently, the hospital in Lake Charles didn't know what I had—just that it was cancer.

I went and saw a gynecologic oncologist. That's the first time I heard "small cell neuroendocrine carcinoma." I had to have her write it down. I was told it was a rare and aggressive cancer and not much was really known about it, but we would fight it aggressively and hope for the best. Honestly, all I heard was ". . . rare and aggressive, blah, blah, blah." Luckily I had someone with me who could pay attention! I was sent to the Willis Knighton Cancer Center and met my radiation oncologist and my chemotherapy oncologist. Of course, I couldn't start treatment till my body was healed from the surgery. Everything was planned for May 2010.

I rented a room in a very sweet old man's house. I was at the hospital in Shreveport at 4 a.m. to have a port placed in my chest. I was transferred to the center where I received radiation and then on to chemo. It was a lot to take in for one day. I was supposed to have radiation five days a week and chemo twice for six weeks. After the first month, I had only been sick a few times, because I had really good meds, but I became incontinent. I started wearing diapers. I started to get weaker, but it was almost over.

Or so I thought.

I ended up having radiation 5 days a week and chemo three times a week for three months, from May through the end of June. I had only rented a room for one month and my funds were low, so I decided I would drive back and forth. A niece of mine would ride with me just in case I got too sick to drive. My day consisted of getting up at 3:30 am and on the road by 4 am for therapy on Monday, Wednesday, and Friday. I had one really bad day where I was at home, sitting on the edge of the couch, when I started crying. I told my family I couldn't do it anymore. I was tired all the time. I was wearing diapers, and if I forgot to take my meds then I was sick. My skin and creases were being burned and blistered. It hurt to have a bowel movement. I'd have to lie down for about 20 minutes after I had one and let the burning stop. I now had hemorrhoids. I wanted to stop the treatment. I was reminded that I was strong. I was handling this better than anyone thought, and I'm no quitter. I finished treatment with more physical problems than when I just had cancer!

In September, I had a clean PET scan. I beat cancer! I was informed, though, that this type of cancer was wicked, and although I was cancer-free today, it would come back. I currently take 20 mg. of Paxil', which I'll be on forever, if it's up to me! Every time I get a pain, my mind thinks, cancer. My new issues are, when I cough, sneeze, laugh or sometimes just stand up, I urinate. Poise Pads are awesome and I keep diapers for bed time. I've started bleeding when I have bowel movements, this has been going on for a few months but my colonoscopy came back clear so again, doctors don't know what to do. But there is a good side to all of this!

I am no longer scared to live and try new things! I took a class to learn how to ride a motorcycle. I bought one and within a month, I broke my left wrist. I consider it a new experience! I've been on an airplane. Not something I'll do again. I went back to college. I am a 38-year-old freshman going for my bachelor's degree in science to be a nurse. I want to do all the things I should've done when I was younger! I can't have children, but I have the best job ever taking care of a five-year-old boy, a two-year-old girl and a three-month-old baby boy that I got to see come into this world. Another new experience!

No matter what happens to me now, I know I am strong enough to handle it. When new experiences come my way, I jump on them! I sing karaoke with my friends. I eat at new restaurants. I am part of a motorcycle ministry called The Revelators. I quit doing drugs. I read more. I watch more movies. I love more. I'm not afraid. My first bout with cancer has taught me that living life is about the quality of life you live. I have also become "girlie." I was always a jeans and t-shirt kinda gal but now, I still wear my jeans, but I pair them with four inch platform wedges and frilly shirts. I've become more feminine and I like it! I dress better! I quit coloring my hair because I'm proud of my gray! I take better care of my skin and I paint my toenails and fingernails to match. Cancer has been life-changing. I deal with the bad days by dressing up for no reason! I used to go to the store in pajamas if that's what I had on. Not now. I want to be my best at all times. I still have bad days. I still have pain. I am me for the first time in my life!. I no longer try to be what someone else needs me to be. And I love life.

S.—born in 1973 and not dying anytime soon from cancer!

I am 13 ways tough!

Let your mind start a journey through a strange new world.
Leave all thoughts of the world you knew before. Let your soul
take you where you long to be . . . Close your eyes let your spirit
start to soar, and you'll live as you've never lived before.
                                    —*Erich Fromm*

Dave Smyth, Sr.

My name is Dave Smyth, Sr. I live in Port Orchard, Washington. I was born in Vallejo California in 1956 and married in 1974. I have two older brothers and one older sister. My Mom and Dad passed away to a better place in 2010. I have a daughter and a son, both in their early thirties. I started a journal back in August 2008 of events that happened and changed it into a story that I want to share.

I know cancer is not a pain of itself, but it does cause it. Over the years I have been living with a pain that I hid from a lot of people, including myself. It wasn't until July of 2008 that I could not take it anymore. Was I scared, was I stupid, was I selfish, or was I just in plain denial? Why would I have cancer? No one in my family had it. I was expecting some type of other problems over the years like a stroke or a heart attack, but never cancer.

In March of 2000, as I was getting ready two days before a business trip, I became really sick. I lay in bed and my stomach began to swell up. It was so big I could not touch my fingers putting my elbows on my side. My wife and daughter came home and could not find me for a little while. I didn't want to yell out once they found me in bed. I told them I was going to be OK. For two days I could not move. I could not breathe normally nor swallow. The pain—have you ever had someone give you a strong-grip handshake? That is what it was like for twenty four hours a day in my stomach. After a few days, it went away and I was fine for a long time.

In 2006, the same pain and swelling started again. As time went on I would come home from work, knowing that I had a few hours to be alone because my wife would be working at her business. I would come into the house, get up the stairs, and go right to the floor in the living room and lie down. I would stay there until the phone rang or I heard a car door. I'd get up and try to act as if everything was fine. I felt like being sick, but I would have to talk myself out of it and hold it in. Days, weeks, months and years went by with the pain and swelling, and still, I told no one. There was one time when my wife left to go shopping and left me at home. I couldn't wait for her to leave: I had to lie down. She came right back and I went into my garden shed and closed the door. I lay on the floor. I could hear her yell for me and heard her walking around the yard. Again, I didn't want her to know anything was wrong or to see me in pain, so I just lay quietly. She left, and I knew she was upset, because she locked me out of the house. She didn't know about all of this until later on, after things started to happen with me.

Eventually my pain started to show. I made excuses for it—"I just didn't feel good", "Something I ate", "Must be work stress". High blood pressure became an issue, and some excessive medication really helped out my excuses. I even made two trips to Ireland in 2006 and 2008 with my son, following each of his two tours of duty in Iraq. The pain was still there, but it didn't matter: I was with my son. Restrooms became my new best friend.

I was finding that going to the bathroom started to relive some of my pain. It became very painful going, but it was a new pain. I never had any pain pills but I always wished I could get some. I can only describe my new pain as, for a boy or a man, if you were kicked or fell on your private area, that pain . . . all the time: sleep or not, standing or sitting, eating or drinking. That pain started the first part of 2008, and by July, I could not take it any longer.

The Sunday after the 4th of July, 2008, I just could not take it any longer. I finally told my wife and my daughter I needed to see a doctor. Several doctors asked about my pain level, out of ten, ten being the worst. All I could say was I was at a twelve. They asked all the fifty-plus year questions: chest pain, shortness of breath, and so on. I told them I was having a lot of stomach pain. The time finally came to get checked out. Finding out what I had was to be difficult. A battery of tests followed: upper and lower GI scans, blood tests and more. The doctor told me I wasn't going anywhere for a few days. I was having a hard time communicating with the nurses and from what I was told my blood pressure really started to climb, 230/160 and higher. At one time it was at 280/210 and I was really starting to lose it. I called my wife at 3 o'clock in the morning to tell her something was going to happen. But I didn't know what was going to happen.

The next day a surgeon came in to talk with me. He told me he was going to perform an operation to find out what was going on. He said he was going to do it laparoscopically and he would see me later. That night he came in to say he had removed a carcinoid tumor, although he was not able to do it laparoscopically. I had an incision all the way up. I lost my belly-button and it was very different for me. He told me it was cancer, and that there were two spots on my liver that were of interest. He removed several large tumors too. Both my surgeon and oncologist were concerned with the area on my liver. My oncologist told my wife and I that he was classifying my carcinoid cancer as a "Stage Four." I was told my prognosis would be two to five years.

After my staples had been removed, I began a number of tests again. A twenty four urine test, four day nuclear injection scan, blood work, and then I began some treatments. The pain continued. I could not sleep and didn't feel like doing anything. I was depressed. I was fatigued, and didn't know what was going on. Carcinoid syndrome had taken over my life. I started keeping a journal, writing down my thoughts and activities. I went back to work in late August 2008, but it was a trying time for me. November came and I was still in pain. The oncologist said it was time to do a little alternative to chemotherapy. A therapeutic injection was made and another CT Scan. I had a scheduled appointment with my surgeon for the middle of December, but he called me at work and said he wanted to see me right away. He said he really needed to get back in and remove a large mass that was identified by the last CT scan, as well as tumors on my lymph nodes and on my liver. He said if I did not choose to go ahead with surgery, he would be able to give me some medication to relieve some of my pain for the time I had left with my life. I told him I could not deal with this pain any longer, that I wanted to do it. He warned me that there would be some upfront problems, but he was planning to remove all of my small intestines and would put in a small section to connect my stomach to my colon. He also said I would end up with a feeding tube for the rest of my life. I asked if I could hold off until after the holidays and he was ok with that but said he needed to do it as soon as possible.

My second surgery was scheduled for January 7, 2009. The surgeon told my wife that everything went well and he was able to get a lot of the tumors. The problems he had thought he might have did not happen. He removed the large mass and other tumors with it and there would be no feeding tube. He did say, however, that he didn't get all the tumors. Coming out of recovery into my room at the hospital I was asked how I felt. All I could say is I had not felt this good in years. Afterwards though, the pain continued daily, all day and night. It was about an 8 to 10 level all the time. I continued to work the best I could. I returned to my oncologist and told him he needed to do something about the pain. He sent me to a pain specialist who did a surgery to implant an Intrathecal Pain Pump in September 2009.

I had the surgery to implant the pump. From the time I woke up in recovery my pain level was down to a solid two (2). I felt "Great". With the small setback of an infection just over a few weeks, I was still at a "2". I was getting 200 mg. of morphine 24 hours a day. I was referred to a world-renowned carcinoid specialist at the University of Oregon who told me my pancreas was shutting down. In March of 2010, I developed a bad leak in my back where the catheter from the pain pump went into my spine. The pain specialist did another surgery on my back, and, although it stopped leaking, he was a little puzzled. After two weeks it started to leak again. He had to remove the pain pump. I had developed a very bad case of MRSA, and ended up with a PICC line. I had to give myself IV's for 45 days. That medication was Vancomycin, the granddaddy of all for the treatment of infections. After that, it was six weeks of medication. What an experience! During this time, I was taking medication and was still going to work. One morning, while driving to work, I fell asleep and ran off the road and wrecked my car. Fortunately, I didn't hurt myself, but I was just a little shaken up.

I planned to start using my sick leave again and get ready to retire after 37 years. My plan was to retire in March 2011. The remainder of the sick leave I had left allowed me to leave early and continue going to the doctors. I left work the middle of September 2010. The first week out I spent every day at the doctors. I developed jaundice, turning a nice shade of yellow. They could not figure out what was really going on. In the mean time I had made an appointment with the pain specialist again and it was decided to implant another pain pump.

After more testing it was determined that my gallbladder needed to be removed. The doctor had to leave one of the areas open and let it heal from the inside out. Having that was really interesting for my wife. She ended up cleaning that area twice a day for two weeks and she had a hard time with that. That took care of the jaundice.

Three weeks later I went in for another surgery to have the pain pump implanted. I was back to 200 mg. of morphine 24 hours a day. Everything was healing up and I felt great.

Cancer has really changed my life. The Intrathecal Pain Pump has also made a change in my life—a big change. This pain pump has given me a new way of thinking about my cancer. I can deal with it better without so much pain. I just can't believe that one doctor changed my entire life like that. What a lesson learned for me!

Again something new for me started up. Back in April 2012, I had a grand mal seizure, and I ended up in the hospital. I had another in June. A new doctor said he wasn't sure what caused them, but he didn't put me on anti-seizure medication after the first one. After the second seizure, he started me on the medication. It sure plays havoc on me. I can't drive any longer and can't do a lot of things. All my doctors have told me that they don't know if these seizures are associated with or caused by carcinoid.

My wife just turned me on to a carcinoid site on Facebook and shared with me a story about a young lady who just experienced a first-time seizure and they found it to be associated with the placement of her Intrathecal Pain Pump. I'm not too sure what to think about all of that yet. My wife, R. has been very supportive. I could not have gone through all of this without her. A few (very few) friends have been supportive too.

I heard something a while back that when a person is told they have terminal cancer that is all they can think about. You don't know how true that is. I will have to say this: I have heard that cancer changes lives all over. Cancer seems to bring families and friends closer. In my case that has not happened. Not sure why, but it has driven my family and friends apart. It sure hurts. I have a lot to do. I have taken care of most of my business. When I do move on into another place, my wife should not have a lot to take care of. I love and care a lot about my wife and my friends, of the ones that I have. They all mean a lot to me.

I started this carcinoid story shortly after I was diagnosed. I have tried to keep it up to date, and, as you have read, I have changed over the months. I think the medication plays a lot with my mind. Some days I have a really hard time remembering things. Not too sure what is going to happen over the next day, weeks, months, or years. I hope to continue living and fulfilling my dreams!

Richard "Spike" Redding

My story

I was born in 1946, one of the many children born into the group known as the "Baby Boomers". I had a normal childhood growing up as an "Army brat".

In 1958 my mother was diagnosed with breast cancer. She had a bilateral mastectomy. This was her only treatment. She died last year after having been diagnosed with a second primary cancer of the lung. She was treated in 2010 with chemotherapy and radiation. In March of 2012 she was diagnosed with a metastasis of her lung cancer to the brain. She was treated with radiation and sadly, she died in August of the same year at age ninety one.

My Father was diagnosed with colon cancer in 1961 and had no treatments but required a colostomy. He died in 1962 of a possible metastasis to the liver.

In 1965 I joined the United States Army and went to Vietnam in 1967 to 1968. It was there I was exposed to Agent Orange.

I was honorably discharged from the Army in 1969 and married a year later. At this time I rejoined the Army.

In 1975 my son Joshua was born, and in 1977 along came my second son Matthew.

I left the Army in 1981 after a total of fourteen years of active duty. I became a Health-Physics technician at Rancho Seco Nuclear Generation Station near Sacramento, California.

In 1992 I started to have pains in my lower abdomen, sharp, intense and intermittent. My diet changes helped but the pain persisted and eventually I started to have bouts of diarrhea.

This would go on for two to three days and I had to stay close to bathrooms. It did not seem to be connected to the abdominal pain.

I informed my family physician about my symptoms in 1993. He ordered blood tests and the results were insignificant. After several more bouts of this pain he ordered an upper and lower gastrointestinal series. This too, was non revealing. Eventually my doctor ordered a colonoscopy. An internist performed the study and took a biopsy of a suspicious sight. The results came back as "atypical cells". I was told I might have Crohn's disease. The doctor who performed the colonoscopy knew about carcinoid, and therefore, the tissue sample was tested for carcinoid and indeed, I received a diagnosis of "carcinoid cancer". I also had a twenty-four-hour urine test (5HIAA) and serum serotonin, and these were high, lending credence to the biopsy results.

At this point I was relieved that I did not have Crohn's disease. I feel that cancer can be cured, because both my parents had cancer and survived. I was advised to see a surgeon to have the carcinoid removed. I talked with the surgeon and he told me it was a simple surgery to remove the tumor. While he was exploring my insides during the surgery, he informed me that he would make sure that he got the entire tumor out and check for other abnormalities.

I had surgery in August of 1993 and several weeks later, after my recovery, my surgeon told me what he had done. He removed my ascending colon and about eighteen inches of small intestine. This was probably my primary tumor. He also removed lymph nodes from this region because of metastasis.

My surgeon then performed an ultrasound of my liver and found fourteen more tumors. He was able to remove ten of the biggest ones but left the others because they were small and he could remove them in about five years if they grew.

His advice was "go home and have a good time, enjoy your life, you have nothing to worry about."

In 1995 my wife asked me for a divorce, stating that "I do not want to watch you die."

In 1999 I married again. During our courtship, I was very upfront with my wife about my medical problems as I did not want to hide anything from her. She loved me enough to not stop her from marrying me. We have been married fourteen years.

In 2000 my blood work showed an increase in serotonin levels. It was at this point when my surgeon said that he felt it was time to remove the tumors that had been left in my liver in 1993. I had cryo-ablation on the remaining tumors. He removed four tumors but noticed many small tumors that were distributed throughout my liver. He said they resembled tapioca.

At this point the surgeon advised me to see an oncologist and that I had eighteen months to live.

I went to see an oncologist and he started me off with three rounds of 5FU chemotherapy. This was followed by daily interferon injections and monthly Sandostatin LAR* injections at sixty milligrams.

My wife and I looked for a support group and found a small group that met once a month in Roseville, California. It was started by J. S., since deceased, after she herself had recently been diagnosed with Carcinoid cancer. We found out there was not much information on how to treat Carcinoid cancer, and there were few doctors who even knew how to treat carcinoid patients. We found out about patient seminars around the country and started attending them. To date we have gone to eight or nine of these conferences.

In 2001 I was diagnosed with type II diabetes and started daily injections of insulin.

My brother died of esophageal cancer in 2002 after serving two tours in Vietnam. He was never evaluated for exposure to Agent Orange.

After a consultation with an oncologist at UCSF, I was advised to stop my interferon. He felt it was not very efficacious and may have lead to my renal failure.

My serotonin levels rose again in 2006. At this point my surgeon suggested Radio Frequency Ablation (RFA) on the liver tumors and attempted to remove my gallbladder as a preventive measure as octreotide can cause gallstones. He attempted to remove the gallbladder via laparoscope, but was unable to and I had open surgery. He performed RFA on several of the liver tumors then suggested I have chemoembolization the next day. I agreed with this plan and had the procedure. I was discharged two days later, with the expectation of having another chemoembolization done in several months.

Two months later I went into kidney failure and had to go on dialysis for several weeks.

During a routine CT scan of my abdomen and pelvis, a spot was found on my left kidney. A biopsy revealed renal cell carcinoma. The surgeon performed RFA on the tumor to remove it. I am very fortunate it was found early.

I had another episode of kidney failure in 2011 and went on dialysis three times a week, from July to November. My kidneys recovered enough that I was able to stop dialysis. While undergoing dialysis one of the nurses suggested that since I am a veteran I apply to the Veterans Administration for benefits. I submitted my paperwork to the VA for my medical conditions. After several months of testing and interviews, the VA determined that I was eligible for benefits and classified my disability as service connected. I was rated 100% disabled. This was traced back to possible Agent Orange exposure in Vietnam.

I applied for a clinical trial for a Ga68 (Gallium scan) in 2012 and was told that I did not qualify because of my underlying kidney problems.

To this day I remain on thirty milligrams of Sandostatin LAR® every twenty eight days. I don't know the full extent of my disease at this time. Now that the initial clinical trials are over I may be able to get a Ga68 scan this year. This will give me a better picture of what is going on with my cancer.

Out of all this experience I have learned that I have be an advocate for my health. I work with my local doctors to get the treatments I need. I have to constantly educate them and their staff on new and changing ideas on the treatment of NETs. I have at times had to plead my case with the medical insurance company to seek advice and treatment outside my local area. I have been accepted after a lengthy process of appeal.

Are my health problems a result of exposure to Agent Orange in Vietnam? I don't know. The VA says that my diagnosis of Diabetes is recognized as being caused by this exposure. However, they don't think that NETs have a direct correlation to Agent Orange.

I continue to work with the Northern California CarciNet (NCCN) Support Group. They have put on several mini-seminars, and also have support group meetings every other month. NCCN is a great resource for information and also the support from other members in the group helps me and my wife in battling NETs.

I find other activities to keep me from always thinking about carcinoid, but it is always in the back of my mind and can rear its ugly head at any time.

I have come to believe that there is no expiration date for me. Life is about being born and we all will die. No one escapes from leaving this plane.

Be bold and mighty forces will come to your aid."
—Basil King

Anna Haslam

My journey with carcinoid began in February 2010 when I was packing in readiness to move out of my home. I kept getting a sudden, right sided, sharp pain just below my rib cage. It lasted only a few minutes and was gone as quickly as it started. I have had several para-umbilical and epigastric hernia repairs; therefore, I automatically assumed that due to all the packing and lifting, I had strained myself and, in the process, acquired another hernia.

I sold up, moved house, and by August 2010 the pains were coming a little more frequently. I knew I would have to address the possibility of yet more surgery, which I had wanted to avoid. I saw my general practitioner for another matter and casually mentioned this new pain.

On examination, my doctor told me she had found a mass and it wasn't a hernia, because hernias don't occur in that region of the torso. By now I was also having bouts of unusual, putrid-smelling diarrhea on a daily basis and feeling really hot (flushing) within ten minutes of eating or drinking anything, including water. Small amounts of alcohol were one of the worst offenders to cause these symptoms.

I was referred on a two-week urgent appointment to a bowel consultant, whom I saw mid-September. He examined me and also confirmed he could feel this mass and referred me for an urgent CT scan. Two weeks later the scan showed two possible polyps and what looked like some fecal matter trapped in my appendix. My consultant than decided a colonoscopy was required.

I had the colonoscopy in the latter part of October. I was awake for the procedure, except for mild sedation. The colonoscopy took an hour and fifteen minutes to complete. No polyps were found but I could see, on the camera screen, something in my appendix. It appeared to be a tumor of some kind. It looked grey and was saucer shaped and attached to the side of the appendix. It protruded slightly into my large bowel. Not many people can say that they have looked inside their bowels!

The consultant was able to look into my small intestine and pronounced it as looking healthy. He took biopsies of the tumor for further analysis. He then informed me he needed to remove the appendix and possibly part of my large intestine and had to do this pretty swiftly! The lab results came back a couple of weeks later as benign. I was so relieved!

My operation date was set for Friday, December 10th, 2010. I was told my surgeon intended to remove my appendix by laparoscope technique and would also perform an ileocecal re-section. I went down to the surgical theatre at 1:40 p.m. and was due back on the ward by 5:00 p.m. Things didn't go quite as planned, however. Although the surgeon tried using a laparoscope, due to my previous hernia repairs I had a lot of mesh in my stomach and this, unfortunately, made it difficult to reach the area. I was opened up with a large incision instead. I did not return to the ward until almost 10 p.m. My surgeon did an incredible job. My poor family, meanwhile, were understandably terribly concerned by my late return to the ward!

During the five weeks since the colonoscopy, the tumor had grown at quite an alarming rate into my large bowel and my appendix was on the verge of bursting. My pains had certainly become more frequent prior to my operation.

I was terribly sick following surgery. My discomfort continued for twelve days despite anti-nausea drugs. Due to the two operative procedures to open me up I was black and blue down the entire side of my left torso around to my spine and down my right thigh. Every time a doctor examined me he/she commented that they had never seen anything quite like it! My bowels were completely out of control as well. I was incontinent and due to the persistent vomiting my throat and mouth were full of ulcers and blisters. I was very ill, no pretending here. I found eating almost impossible for those first few weeks. Apart from the nausea and vomiting I was in a great deal of pain too. I was discharged from hospital fourteen days following my surgery. My consultant had wanted to keep me in longer, but, alas, an infectious diarrheal episode had broken out on the ward and that was the last thing he wanted me exposed to. I was, therefore, discharged to home.

I was awaiting the ambulance to take me home when suddenly my consultant reappeared and asked to see me in a private room. It was in this room I discovered and heard for the first time that I had "carcinoid cancer". The biopsy results from the bowel surgery had in fact shown carcinoid in a few of the lymph nodes as well. I was told the tumor was benign as originally thought. My surgeon further explained that my tumor was like a cancer, but not really a cancer and there was no treatment except to find it early and cut it out. Chemotherapy and radiotherapy were apparently not options as weapons against this dreadful disease. He said "It may never return. It may return within a year, or two or five; or some patients had even lived as long as twenty years following their initial diagnosis." I would have annual CT scans to check for any new growths.

For months following surgery, I had to stay home while I tried to regain control of my bowels. The sensation of needing a bowel movement was gone. I had to try and pre-guess the need for a visit to the bathroom. I veered between liquid movements to constipation. I can only describe this as going into the operating theatre with my bowels and feeling as if I had come out with someone else's!

Foods that I used to like and enjoy, I could no longer tolerate. Salads and meat induced terrible pain as they passed through my system. I was still experiencing bouts of flushing following meals and even when drinking water. Eating or drinking also induced the most horrific heartburn. I was living on Gaviscon! Over the months the flushing improved, but has never really disappeared.

My annual CT scan in December 2011 showed a new growth on my liver. There was a cyst on my left lobe measuring approximately 4 to 5 cm. This time I was referred to an oncologist who authorized a 5-HIAA urine test and a fasting gut hormone blood test. She gave me printouts to help me read about carcinoid on the internet. There is not as much information as I would like out there, and I am also discovering there are very few doctors here in the U.K who specialize in carcinoid cancer.

In February 2012, I was also sent for a special liver MRI scan with contrast. The results returned, and, once again, I was told this new tumor was a benign cyst.

Throughout the summer of 2012, I have been suffering from abnormal heart rhythms, an increase in flushing, breathlessness and on occasion, the horrid—smelling diarrhea. This month my oncologist saw me again and assured me I am cured! However, she has authorized another 5-HIAA urine collection test and another fasting gut hormone. I am currently awaiting the results of these tests.

I am so grateful to be alive, but I have altered my lifestyle. These days I avoid chocolate and barely touch alcohol, except for a rare glass of wine. I endeavor to avoid foods that are from the nightshade family. This will not cure me, but I do try to make my body's environment as hostile as possible to cancer. I also avoid caffeinated drinks or fizzy drinks. Going out involves knowing where there is a readily available bathroom and finding foods on the menu that do not upset me. I try to eat mostly vegetables, whole grains, beans, and fruits that agree with me. I find figs, raspberries and blueberries are kind to my system. I also try to eat no more than 500 grams of red meat in a week. This is easily achievable as red meat is still hard for me to digest.

I have found a couple of excellent carcinoid support groups on Facebook and am about to meet another lady here in the U.K who, like me, has carcinoid cancer. I cannot wait to see her to compare notes. Meanwhile, I hope to be one of those patients that has another twenty years in front of them.

Time, as the saying goes, will tell.

> *"Yesterday is history, tomorrow is a mystery, today is a gift of God, which is why we call it the present."*
> —Bil Keane

Wendy Gayle

Pulmonary Carcinoid Tumor

Day of Change

I placed the phone down, knowing something wasn't right. I decided to take a five-minute break from all the hustle and bustle at work. The end of summer was here and the start of the cool fall air was just beginning to break the Memphis heat. I needed to go outside and take a deep breath. I needed air, as my chest wall felt like it was compressed and I felt dizzy.

That of course didn't stop me from wanting a cigarette while I talked to the other building smokers. This time it was different, though. I remember telling J. that "Here I am feeling sick and I was out here smoking another damn cigarette." Internally I was having a huge conflict. I didn't want to be doing it but I had to. I took the last puff, went inside and decided I was feeling too weird to just pass it by. I went to my co-worker who was in her office, and I asked her "Can you take me home?" I remember the look on her face and she said to me, in a strange voice, "Nooo, I am going to call 911." We went back into my office and she called 911 and gave them my medical information. She asked me what meds I was taking and the dosage and relayed it to the dispatcher. The receptionist was important to have near, as she would help facilitate the ambulance drivers. They would take me to the stretcher while the receptionist would call my husband and tell them I was on my way to the hospital.

I was scared.

Nothing in life prepares you for when something goes wrong with you and you have no control over what is about to happen. You can only keep your faith and pray.

Emergency Room Hours

We had arrived at the hospital emergency room. I remember seeing my husband as they opened the ambulance door, and, as the medics wheeled me into the ER, I saw my coworker looking frantic, on the phone. I wanted to say "thank you" to her, but she was on the other side of the door and I couldn't speak to her. I remember the doctors ran a heart test and asked questions about my hospitalization, which had been in 2008. I didn't know why they wanted to know about that particular visit. They then disappeared for two hours and came back to take more x-rays.

That's when the silence settled. Just over an hour later, the emergency room doctor came into the room. He had a concerned look on his face and was very compassionate. "We have been comparing your x-rays to the ones that were on file from 2008. It seems you have a mass or a tumor that has grown in this area of your lung." He pointed to his top left portion of his chest. I must have had fear in my eyes because I remember them watering up and all I could think about was the "C" word. I held on to my husbands' hand. I was scared and even more scared now. Our 25th wedding anniversary would be coming up in the next year.

There was no room in the hospital this time, and I had to wait for a few hours before they could admit me into the ICU. My husband and I looked at each other. We didn't say a word. By two in the morning, the Cardiac ICU was ready and I was being admitted.

More tests were ordered. The X-Ray Summary read: IMPRESSION: Left suprahilar mass with relatively smooth surface texture; lobulated in appearance with peripheral contrast enhancement. This has dramatically increased in size from the prior study and may well be a benign lung mass. It appears that it has at least doubled in size over the last two years. Further evaluation with PET CT is recommended for further evaluation to exclude malignancy. This lesion would be amenable to CT-guided biopsy.

My husband and I were both speechless and didn't know how we felt. Just the night before, my husband and I were holding each other and I said to him jokingly "I wheeze when I hold you, and you have COPD, that's so strange." I had actually been saying that for a couple of years, not even thinking twice about what may be happening inside my body.

We had spent the last three years advocating for patient and patient rights and now I was becoming one of "them" a cancer patient and my husband, my advocate.

First Visit to Lung Doctor Day:

I was discharged from the hospital and was told that I would need to follow up with the "Lung Specialist." This meeting would later be the best and most efficient healthcare team I would meet. What I didn't know was that this was the team that was going to make me become cancer free! My first visit to Dr. S. was a normal lung doctor visit. It consisted of a breathing test, lung function test and yes breathing into a machine to check air mass flow. He gave my husband and I ample time to ask questions, even though we weren't sure what to ask at this point. He then said, quite frankly and outright, "if" the tumor were to be cancer we would discuss treatment options.

It wasn't long after we got home that the family had questions. We only wished we knew the answers right then and there to what they were asking. My daughters' questions were "What does Mom have? "What is going to happen?" I explained to them that all those questions and more would be answered once we knew exactly what we were looking at. We didn't have any answers just yet.

PET SCAN and Biopsy Day:

It was a cool fall morning when I woke up to go to work for a few hours. I didn't want to miss too much time from work, as my job required me to be there every day and stay late. My appointment was for later in the morning and I left work to go to my appointment in the midmorning. I wasn't sure what to expect for my first PET scan and biopsy. To be honest it really wasn't that bad to endure. I think waiting for the results was the worst part. I went to the clinic and had my dye test completed for my PET scan. Then I had to go back up to the hospital to have them take out a sample of my lung tissue for further testing for the biopsy. This was done with a long needle and it was, as I remember, pretty pain free due to the medicine they gave me. Unfortunately we had to wait for the results at our next doctor's appointment which was a week away. During this time we were still feeling numb as everything seemed to be happening so fast. Each week ran into the next and I didn't want to believe that we were going through this. Both T. and I were very active in Patient Rights and Advocacy with patients with cancer. We were now practicing what we preached to so many people. Be an informed patient, know your rights and ask questions.

Second Visit to Lung Doctor:

In Dr. S's office both my husband and I waited in the room. We looked at the medical stuff on the wall and then we would talk a little bit and then there would be silence. We would just stare at each other and think things were going to be fine. We were both uncomfortable because we could tell that this visit would be different. During our last visit the nurse was full of life and humor and cracked jokes. When he came into the room this time and I tried to crack a joke with him, he didn't respond. Usually the nurse would come back with a cute remark. This time the outgoing nurse said nothing and was very serious. I could tell the news of the biopsy was news we were not ready to hear. My husband kept telling me to be optimistic and not to worry. About five minutes later Dr. S came into the room. I remember looking at my husband when the news came out of Dr. S's mouth. It was like scenes from a movie where you see the lips slowed down and in slow motion you watch the screen. The lips say in a distorted voice "You, have a rare form of lung cancer."

The doctor was compassionate and truthful. "You are only the 3rd case I have ever seen in my 40 years of practice." He used the term "team", and we were going to work together with a surgeon. Both my husband and I needed to hear we had a strong anchor. We were not sure what we were in for but we all knew "together" was the key.

Dr. S. delivered the news as though he was going to get us through it. We were numb, scared and unsure of what was going to happen. I had one more visit and one more doctor to meet. That surgeon is Dr. E.

The Surgeon

The next critical person on our team was Dr. E, the surgeon. The past month was going by so fast that we simply hadn't had the time to ingest what was happening to us. As both my husband and I remember pulling into the doctor's parking lot, we got out of the car and for a brief moment looked into each other's eyes. I wonder what was going through my husband's mind. I think for the first time we could both say we were never prepared or scripted in life for this type of situation. As we walked into Dr. E's office I saw that the office was full. This is a good sign I thought. A lot of people come to this doctor. Then as I sat down I really started to look at people. Some had foot surgery; others arm surgery. There was an elderly man whose leg had been amputated. As I sat in the office waiting for them to call us back, I made eye contact with a woman. She asked "hey, what are you here for? You seem too young to be here. Look at us", as she pointed around the room. I told her I had a tumor in my lung; carcinoid lung cancer. She told me I was with one of the best doctors in Memphis. While we waited for Dr. E's nurse to call us back to the patient area, I watched how the room emptied out as patients were being seen. Finally, we were called back to a room. Dr. E., who kind of reminded me of Robin Williams in Patch Adams, came into the room. His personality was so warm; I gave him my trust right away. He came in with a plan and he had obviously researched my records because he was ready with any questions we had for him. My first question was "how do you take the lung out?" He answered there are two ways to do this, either through your armpit, as he lifted up his arm, or through your shoulder and he pointed behind my back and rubbed the shoulder blade area. He did say that his plan was to extract the upper left lobe where the tumor was. That way there wouldn't be any chance for the tumor recurring in the lung. Originally I had thought they would do an incision like open-heart surgery in the front to take my lung out, so I was relieved. I wouldn't want to see the scar every day on the front of my body. I was kind of relieved that the extraction took place in the back, mainly so I wouldn't be reminded of the cancer. Later I would find out that all that thinking was so wrong, and the healing would take a couple of years. After listening to Dr. E we now had a plan and my medical team was in order.

There was so much to get done now that we knew what was going to happen in a couple of weeks. There would be phone calls to loved ones and friends and I would set up a family meeting with my daughters. Both of them were so strong and helped me through this trying time. Of course, they had questions about what "the plan" was and my husband and I were able to answer them to the best of our ability.

There was a quiet time when I asked my daughter to have her name on the Advance Directive paperwork. I told her my wishes and asked that if something unforeseen happened, she would be strong enough to follow through with them. Luckily, no measures were needed. I explained that it was important to talk about Advance Directives and that you don't need to have surgery to have your wishes on paper. An Advance Directive insured one's wishes were met. Even to this day we have our Advance Directives in the safe.

R. and I would also be online and she would reach out for support from her friends during this time. This was also the time where I would be reading and searching for people who had my same problem. This is when I found great people on Facebook in the Carcinoid Coffee Cafe and an online support group for Carcinoid Cancer.

The Day of Surgery

Both my husband and I were up and down all night long. By the time the alarm clock rang we were just laying there in bed watching the ceiling fan spin. We were already worn out from the anticipation of what was going to happen. I remember that it was a quiet morning. We looked at each other and knew what had to be done. We readied and drove to the hospital. We checked into the hospital and I was prepped for surgery. The last thing I remember when being wheeled into the operating room was country music playing and Dr. E. telling the nurse that the radio station was fine. The next thing I knew, I was awake and in ICU.

During the week previous, I had called and asked my husband's sister M. if she would come up to help support T. during this time. Naturally, T. stayed at the hospital ICU until I was discharged. Knowing that his sister was going to be there when I came home from the hospital was a God send. One would think that after having a lobe of your lung removed you would heal slowly. This was not the case. She was surprised to know I was sitting up and walking around a few days after major surgery.

To be honest, the first few days were a bear. ICU was like boot camp. Having to breathe in these tubes and having slight

185

complications made me hate this phase of healing. But I had to remind myself I was now cancer free and healing.

My daughters R. and J. came in to see me and to support their dad. They proudly wore these beautiful ribbons that had the Zebra print on them. R. had been into arts and crafts and had found a website that had the zebra print ribbons. They also had made some for the nurses to wear so they could bring awareness to carcinoid cancer. I remember one nurse saying, "This is a teachable moment."

When I returned home I found get well cards from all over the country. My daughter and her friends and family were letting us know we were in their prayers.

Looking back

It has been 2 years since I had the surgery. I have healed and looking at me, you would never guess that I had carcinoid cancer or have the upper lobe of my lung missing. I have to say that during these past two years each month has been a blessing as I have healed almost 100%.

One of the best blessings I have had during the past two years was when we decided that we wouldn't go to Scotland in October for our 25th wedding anniversary. Instead of dreaming about "doing" in life we were going to live our dreams and we, therefore, decided to buy our dream dogs. Little did I know that I would soon learn the value added to life by Sir and Lady. These dogs seemed to have a healing balm about them. This was true for me, but also for everyone we seemed to meet. I brushed them with my left arm to exercise the muscles and later when walking used the left arm to help build strength. My grandchildren would love on them and found that training them was fun and it was somehow therapeutic to have these dogs around to love on. People always stopped us to tell us their stories of their bullies or bassets. We loved hearing their stories and wouldn't have heard about them or met these people if we didn't have Sir and Lady.

Today we don't take the fastest route anywhere. We take the scenic route. We appreciate everyone and everyplace we travel to or meet when shopping.

Having had this experience and being told by all the doctors "everything was a best case scenario" is a blessing. We will continue to advocate for patients with cancer. I used to do it in memory of my parents who both died of cancer. Now I do it for those that are also survivors of cancer.

People look at me and say "But you look so good, it's hard to believe you had cancer." I can only contribute this to my medical team and family and friends. I have been blessed. Some say I have an angel watching over me.

Thank you for letting me share my story with you.

> *Hope is the thing with feathers*
> *That perches in the soul*
> *And sings the tune without the words*
> *And never stops at all.*
> —*Emily Dickinson*

Lynda

I never really had what I would call symptoms. I am a walking example of why ones goes for a routine colonoscopy. I was having some issues with a hemorrhoid and went to my doctor for that reason. I had put off my colonoscopy for a year but for some reason felt it was time to go this time. I usually get nervous when I am going to have tests, but this time I just kept moving forward with it. On April 18, 2012, I had my first colonoscopy.

Afterward, my doctor told me she found a lesion in my ileum. I work with her, so I asked if she felt it was cancer. She said she did think it was but to wait for the pathology report. From that day forward, it became what I like to call the "cancer roller coaster". I went for my blood work, CT and octreotide scans. The day of the CT scan, I was scared to death of what was going to be found. I cried my way through the study. The results came back and my doctor called and stated that the tumor was on the outside of my intestine with lymph node activity. No other tumors were seen.

My doctor then referred me to a surgical oncologist. I met with him a month after my diagnosis. He told me that he wanted me in surgery in a week. He was worried that I would get sicker and did not want to wait. I had plans to go to Hawaii for a family reunion in a month and I was well enough to go.

I had ileo-colostomy surgery on May 29th. My surgeon said I did well and explained that lymph nodes were removed for further analysis and he would inform me of the results in a week. I was in the hospital for one week. I went to see him a week later and was told that the tumor was a well-differentiated NET. I had nineteen lymph nodes removed and nine were positive for cancer. One of the lymph nodes was outside the margins.

I did not know what to do with all this overwhelming information. My sister was with me throughout my ordeal, and my brother also came from his home town for the surgery and support. I also have an 18-year-old son. All have been very supportive, as I undergo the changes this cancer has brought into my life.

I was scared throughout this experience, to say the least. I work as a patient advocate and have been in health care all my life. It was very different to be on the other side now: the one needing help. I also realize that I have a full life to be lived and am willing to be helped to get to that goal.

I went to see an oncologist, but he and I were not compatible. The information he gave me was correct, but the way he acted made me feel like I was just another patient, and he did not agree with my surgeon's proposed next steps. I walked out of that office. I did not want to be a rare cancer patient that would just be forgotten. My surgeon is incredible and felt that I might be a good candidate for Sandostatin˙ shots, but he said that many doctors might not agree. I went to another oncologist who was more on board with me and was willing to work with my surgeon.

Dr. Gannon, from the start, told me that I would meet doctors that would tell me, "Oh you have carcinoid cancer, that is the good kind". He said it was not true. I have heard that quite a few times since my diagnosis.

I am new to the cancer world, as it has only been 4 months since diagnosis. Next month I will receive another CT scan and blood work, which will be the norm for me now. I have always believed there is a positive for a negative, so I plan on taking the day off for my test and treating myself to a massage.

I am still scared of my future. This cancer has changed a lot of what I did and who I was, but it has also allowed me to see how precious life is; how short it can be. I am a 51-year-old, very young and healthy person.

The good that has come and will continue to come out of this experience is that I now live each day to the fullest. I no longer say no to going out and go if I can. I am still learning about this cancer and what to ask. I sometimes feel like I am not as sick as others, so I should not complain or take advantage of services that are offered to cancer patients. But I am a cancer patient, and a very lucky one at that! I plan on having a fund raiser in April, a year after my diagnosis. This positive plan was suggested by my sister and I want the money we raise to go into research for this cancer.

My sister has been there for me all along. I love her more for that, even though I know she is scared for me at times. I have a huge group of friends of all ages who have helped me—from making me dinners, to just calling to check on me.

I am feeling well overall, but sometimes I do get depressed but try to move past it. I aim to create a stress-free life and enjoy it to the fullest. I have trouble with food at times with stomach and bowel issues which can be frustrating.

Even though I have these physical and mental issues, which are normal for someone with cancer, I appreciate my life even more and vow to continue to live my life to the fullest.

At the time of this publication, I am going in for my routine tests and a colonoscopy to see if there have been any changes in my status.

The very least you can do in your life is figure out what you hope for. And the most you can do is live inside that hope. Not admire it from a distance but live right in it, under its roof.
—Barbara Kingsolver, Animal Dreams

Sharon

It Could Be Worse . . .

I'm forty nine years old! I can't believe I'm almost fifty! I am a divorced woman. I was married for eleven years and have no children.

I have one dog and I'm down to one horse. I had two, but sold one to help pay for my medical expenses. I've loved horses since I can remember. My mom said the first words out of my mouth were, "I want a horse!" I finally bought one when I was twenty six, but that is another story.

My parents both died from cancer. My mother's first cancer was lung and later, colon cancer appeared in her ileum, ironically in the same place as mine. After surgery for her colon cancer, my mother opted to not have chemotherapy again. The chemotherapy for her lung cancer really wiped her out and she said she just couldn't do it again. She died from metastatic liver cancer a few years later; a metastasis from her intestinal cancer to the liver. My father passed away after also refusing any follow-up treatment for his rectal cancer. Both my parents were over 70 when they were diagnosed with colon cancer. We feel that my father had his cancer for years before he was diagnosed.

I had my first screening colonoscopy on June 14th, 2012, after my yearly checkup with my Nurse Practitioner. We made a decision that I might as well get the exam over with based on my family history. I didn't expect it to be more than a routine exam. When I woke up, I was in a great deal of pain and very nauseated. Medication eased my pain and I got dressed, ready to go home. When the gastroenterologist came in, he sat down and told me he had found a large mass in my small intestine which was too big for him to remove and that I would need surgery. He said he'd biopsied it but didn't think it looked cancerous. He told me I would need a CT scan and some blood work. The studies were scheduled for the next day. They also gave me an appointment to see a surgeon the following week. At this point, I wasn't too worried as I'd had other tumors removed. They turned out to be fatty and benign. One of the tumors was in my hip, and I also had a breast biopsy. I continue to have a tumor in my lower leg that I've had for thirty years.

I had my CT scan and blood work the day after my colonoscopy, on a Friday. On Monday, the doctor called me and said "I'm so sorry but you do have cancer and its spread to your liver". What? He said I had over 20 tumors in my liver—from several millimeters to 3 centimeters, but that some of them might be benign hemangiomas. I was devastated and in shock, to say the least. I was especially shocked to be given this news as it was delivered to me over the phone while at work! I will say that the doctor seemed somewhat appalled to be giving me this news. I wish he would have called and had me come in to get the bad news in person, even if I did not expect bad news. He went on to tell me it was carcinoid cancer, a rare, slow-growing type. He asked me when I was going in to see the surgeon and felt that it was good I was going soon.

I have lived with my oldest sister since moving back to the state when I got divorced. She's been awesome to me and would give me the shirt off her back. For some reason I didn't tell her that the doctor had called me and told me I had cancer. I'm not really sure why. I've always been a "do it myself" kind of gal, and I just didn't tell her! In hind-sight, I should have told her immediately. She would have helped me research it more that night and she would have come with me to meet the surgeon. Instead I went by myself.

I met the surgeon the next day. I was nervous but wanted to get surgery scheduled, as my insurance was changing in two weeks! He was very nice and seemed very knowledgeable about carcinoid cancer. He said I would have a right hemicolectomy and that they could do it via laparoscope if possible. They would remove part of my ileum, part of the small intestine, and my appendix. I had my gallbladder removed in 2000 or that would have been removed as well. He showed me the CT scan and my liver looked pretty bad to me. Since the tumors were scattered throughout my liver, he could not/would not try and remove them. He said there wasn't a surgeon in our entire state that would! He did tell me that there were surgeons out there who would do it and that it would make my liver look like Swiss cheese! This frightened me! However, I have since learned that there are carcinoid cancer specialists that do surgically remove liver tumors and that it can increase your life expectancy by many years. I learned that they don't even have to get them all, 70 to 90% and it helps quality of life. They do indeed, call it "Swiss cheese" surgery, by the way. Another thing my surgeon told me was that there was a chance I had both carcinoid and colon cancer as my CEA level was high (a blood marker for Duke's colon cancer). This scared me more than anything because I knew that if this was what was in my liver, I wouldn't have too long to live. My mom was gone in three weeks from the time they told her there was nothing they could do for her and about six months from the onset of her symptoms. I never told anyone that this was a possibility. I guess I was in denial and scared!

My surgeon was also concerned about carcinoid crisis during surgery so he wanted me to do a twenty four hour urine test called a 5HIAA. I feel lucky that he knew enough about carcinoid cancer to be concerned, since so many doctors and surgeons seem to know nothing. The results of the test were very high.

I now say that if I'd known then what I know now, I would have waited on the surgery and gone to a specialist out-of-state that could have possibly removed the tumors in my liver at the same time as the right hemicolectomy. I am still kicking myself for that, but I just didn't know!

I had my surgery on July 2, 2012. They removed part of my small intestine, colon and appendix. I actually had eleven tumors in all. Ten were in the small intestine and one in the appendix. Eleven of thirteen lymph nodes were positive for cancer. Biopsies of two of the tumors in my liver were taken.

I do not have colon cancer! It is technically now called well-differentiated neuroendocrine carcinoma, mid-grade, or G2. My Ki-67 was 4%. This test shows the rate of cell mitosis, or growth. I believe its mid-grade just because of the distant metastases but there are still some things I have yet to learn about this cancer.

My recovery was uneventful. I got to watch a wild Fourth of July fireworks show from my hospital room. It was great! I spent only four days in the hospital. I was so glad to get home. My last hospital stay was twenty years ago when I broke my leg and had to have surgery. I think I was there for four days as well. This must be my magic number!

A week after I was discharged from hospital, I had my first appointment with my oncologist. I took my sister with me, as I had many questions and put her in charge of making sure I asked them all. It's so important to take someone with you as all this new information can be so overwhelming. My oncologist is very knowledgeable about carcinoid. He answered all my questions and scheduled me for some additional blood work and an OctreoScan™. We talked about different treatment plans. He too, told me that liver surgery was not an option. He did mention chemoembolization, SIR-spheres* and Thera-Spheres.*

After my OctreoScan™, I went back in and met with the oncologist. He asked me what I wanted to do. That's one of the frustrating things about this cancer, that there didn't seem to be a standard protocol on what to do next. I do not like that I was asked what I wanted done next: I should have been told what would be done next!

I knew I wanted to start on Sandostatin˙ since that is one of the "standards" of treatments. My O-Scan did show positive uptake on some of the tumors in my liver but not all lit up. I'm still not sure what that means, but the Sandostatin˙ should stop the ones that were positive from producing serotonin. I had my first shot that day. It lasts 28 days. It has stopped my diarrhea and my heart palpitations have mostly stopped. I still get them when I'm stressed, however. I am going to ask for the subcutaneous Sandostatin˙ for emergency shots as backup injections for my monthly one. I've learned that we should all have them on hand in case of an emergency. This, sadly, is something my oncologist did not tell me! One really has to research this cancer as there is so much information out there. I wonder if doctors keep up with it since they may only be treating a very small number of patients with carcinoid.

The hardest part now is the waiting. I've heard specialists call this the "wait and worry" plan. Boy, that is so true!

I have taken a huge step forward: Two friends of mine who work in the medical field have both told me about a local liver surgeon who started the liver transplant program here. One of these friends is actually an anesthesiologist, and she works with this doctor. She gave his physician assistant my number, and she called me. He has done many, many liver debulking surgeries on carcinoid patients. He even gets referrals from surrounding states. The bad thing: he's not on my insurance plan for coverage, so his office is trying to get approval for me to go and see him. I have an appointment next week so hopefully they will approve it for at least a second opinion. I'm not sure I will have another major surgery right now, but at least I can talk to him about my options.

I've been thinking about the past ten years or so and wonder if I've had other symptoms that might have pointed to my carcinoid diagnosis. I think I had a few. Diarrhea is the biggest one, but since I had my gallbladder out in 2000, I assumed that it was related to not having my gallbladder. I never really discussed it with any of my doctors, and I'm not sure why. I guess I thought it was normal after gallbladder removal. I didn't have uncontrollable diarrhea: I didn't have twenty bowel movements a day like I hear some have. My diarrhea consisted mostly of loose stools. However, about five years ago, I started to have small, stringy stools. I knew that this could be a sign of something, but I did nothing about it. I don't know why I didn't immediately tell my doctor. I also got really sick after my mother died ten years ago this coming November. I'd eat and then get terrible pain and sometimes throw up. I stopped eating, as it didn't hurt if I didn't eat! I did go to the doctor, but I went as I had a bad upper respiratory infection, and, it turned out to be viral-induced asthma. Asthma can be misdiagnosed carcinoid of the lung, but mine was true asthma. I did tell him about my stomach pain and he ordered an endoscopy. His nurse wanted me to have a colonoscopy when I told her that both my parents had colon cancer, but the doctor thought I could wait. Also, my insurance at the time wouldn't even pay for a screening colonoscopy! I wish I had done it though, but who knows, it may have not shown anything. The EGD (endoscopy) was normal and two days after I had it, I woke up and felt fine. Just like that, my symptoms were gone! I have had similar bouts over the years, but never as bad as the initial ones. The pain then, lasted only a few days to a couple of weeks. I now believe that these symptoms were from the tumors in my small intestines. After my surgery, my surgeon told me that he was shocked I hadn't had a complete obstruction! I think having such loose stools saved me from one. Obviously, a complete obstruction would have revealed my carcinoid cancer sooner.

No one knows what the future will hold. I'm planning on seeing a specialist, but I'm not sure when or which one. I'll have follow-up blood work and some kind of scan in November. I'm anxiously awaiting that day! I try not to dwell on my cancer but honestly, it is all I think about. I try so hard not to, but it's like not thinking about that pink elephant in my living room! I still do research online and check in daily with on-line support groups. I've learned so much from my fellow "noids". My new motto is "it could be worse"!

My family consists of two older sisters, nieces, and nephews (and some darling great-nieces and nephews). My oldest sister is my rock and she is very supportive. I know she would walk through fire for me! That is the type of person she is. My other sister lives several hours away, but I know she's there for me as well. I'm worried about her as she has a disease called "pernicious anemia". It is a blood disorder in which the body can't store or produce vitamin B$_{12}$. People with this disease are more prone to get carcinoid cancer in their stomachs. I've talked with her about it and she is going to have her stomach scoped (EGD) and have a colonoscopy soon. I try not to talk about my cancer too much with the sister I live with. I don't want to overwhelm her or make her "sick" of hearing about it! I fear that that is what she will think. I know it is just me though, because I will be reading something and ask her if she wants to hear it. She always says, "Yes".

I guess I have answered my own question about her love for me!

At this time, February, 2013, I have decided to have the tumors in my liver surgically removed. I will be having this surgery on February 24th. I know I will be alright and with the support of my loving relatives, friends and support groups, I feel more at ease that all will be well!

I am currently recovering from my surgery!(March1st, 2013)

> *There is nothing that wastes the body like worry, and one who has any faith in God should be ashamed to worry about anything whatsoever.*
>
> —Mahatma Gandhi

Howard C. Anderson

My Caregiver Experience

Susan, my wife, doesn't wait for anyone to "give" her care. She actively seeks it out. Therefore, I'm not sure I qualify as a "caregiver". I can describe how her illness affected me and that might be relevant to other "caregivers".

We had been married for 17 years before I ever saw her throw up; summer of 1987. We were driving to a site up in the mountains in Arizona. I think we had eaten hamburgers and I thought maybe she somehow got car-sick due to the gravel road we were traveling on. I had no idea that this was the first indication of a very serious problem and that it would take another 8 years to obtain a diagnosis.

The next eight years (1987 through 1995) were punctuated by emergency room and hospital visits to clear intestinal blockages and attempts to determine the source of the problem. The blockages would typically clear, she would be discharged, and we would hope that maybe it wouldn't happen again.

In 1994, I bought a 10" telescope. I had been interested in Astronomy from the age of 8 but never could afford anything bigger than the one-inch telescope my parents got me for Christmas when I was 10. Finally having a telescope helped me cope with all that was happening in our lives.

Light pollution, even in Arizona, means that to see anything worthwhile, you have to drive at least 50 miles from town. Susan encouraged me to drive the motor home out into the desert so I could do astrophotography even when she was not feeling well enough to come along. In the past, we had always done these sorts of things together. I have always disliked going anywhere without her and without her encouragement I would not have gone.

She eventually had gall bladder surgery and we thought that the problem had finally been resolved. The doctor forgot to come tell me that they had completed the procedure and that she was okay, so I was pretty panicked after three hours with no word. After the surgery, there was some improvement but it was short-lived.

The doctors were involved through regular appointments every three to four weeks although she gradually got worse. They ran many tests, including a liver biopsy, and various blood tests, in an effort to discover what was wrong. No one thought to do a serotonin test even though I mentioned that she turned "lobster red" on occasion.

She accompanied me on business to England. I worked while she took trains and busses and toured England even though she was suffering significant and unrelenting abdominal pain.

We are each other's best friend so it was difficult for me to adjust to her gradually worsening condition. It was so gradual that as we slowly transitioned to keeping her alive exclusively on Dairy Queen Milkshakes, the only thing she could hold down, it almost seemed normal. In a period of 6 months, November 1994 to May 1995, her weight dropped from 160 pounds to 98. The last month she was lying on the couch moaning in pain most of the time. Neither of us thought that the doctors would be able to find anything so she just toughed it out. When she reached 98 pounds, it suddenly dawned on me that this was becoming critical and, if it continued, she would surely die. The doctors, so far, had been unable to find anything to explain her signs and symptoms Therefore, in May, 1995 I concluded that we must become more determined in our efforts to find out why Susan was so ill. We again conferred with the doctor and he suggested enteroclysis.

Enteroclysis involves a tube positioned beyond the stomach valve and liquid is pumped directly into the small intestine so that fluoroscopic imaging can be done. The first indication that they had found something was that the pump slowed down. This indicated some sort of blockage. Surgery then showed that the small intestine was almost completely blocked; narrowed to the size perhaps of a soda straw. The surgeon guessed that it was carcinoid cancer.

When he told me, I think I cried because I was sure she was going to die soon. After having been sick for so long and then to get a cancer diagnosis, to me, meant that it was probably hopeless. They always say cancer can be cured IF YOU TREAT IT EARLY. In this case, it had been going on for 8 years or so! The doctor tried to get me to control my emotions. He thought if she saw me crying that it would have a negative effect on her.

Surprisingly, when I saw her she was much happier about it than I was. She finally had a diagnosis and was already making plans about how to fight the problem! She had me copy the Merck manual pages related to Carcinoid and bring them to her in the hospital. The manual said she'd probably be dead in 2 to 3 years so that didn't help how I felt.

I continued working at Motorola through all this time. I had to make sure we had on-going health insurance. Motorola had an extremely good health insurance plan. We were free to see any doctors anywhere without referral. It was good up to $2 million. (In a Motorola meeting, someone said that after that was exhausted; you should probably make an appointment with Dr. Kevorkian . . .) Motorola has since migrated to another cheaper plan so I guess we were really lucky with respect to timing . . .

When Susan came home, she immediately scoured the internet looking for information on carcinoid. Unfortunately, she found very little. The immediate problem, 33 inches of small intestine containing the primary carcinoid tumor and six lymph nodes had been removed but that was not the full extent of the cancer's infiltration. Liver tumors had been undetected in the Feb 1995 liver biopsy.

She still experienced abdominal pain and diarrhea after the surgery. The abdominal pain was thought to be due to adhesions but we now know it was from additional carcinoid tumors.

It took a couple of more years of research to locate Dr. Warner who, in my opinion, is the reason she is still alive. Dr. Warner prescribed Sandostatin˚ in Feb 1988. In March 1999, Dr. Warner and Susan's local oncologist placed her on Sandostatin LAR˚ and interferon alpha 2b. She says Sandostatin˚ "turned her life around" and gave her a "good quality of life again."

In June 1999, Susan was diagnosed with breast cancer. That is almost a footnote. She again researched everything, did aggressive treatment and, to date, has not had a recurrence.

In October 1999, Susan had a liver resection to eliminate the tumors..A team of five surgeons resected the liver and removed everything else from the abdominal region that looked like or felt like carcinoid. She had earlier received conflicting advice from different doctors regarding whether to do the liver re-section. She again opted for the more aggressive treatment. I am guessing again that she would not be alive now had she not gone ahead with the liver surgery.

I have tried to provide emotional and financial support throughout her ordeal. Currently, my main contribution to her treatment is administering her Sandostatin LAR˚ shot once a month. One of my earliest memories is being in a hospital with pneumonia and receiving penicillin every three hours. When I have to take a blood sample from her, I grit my teeth and look away. I've never watched. However, I have learned to inject her Sandostatin˚. I have figured out how to prevent the needle from clogging. Once, when we were camping, we forgot to bring extra needles so I managed to do the injection without switching needles so I would have the second one for a spare if needed. I hate it when the needle clogs . . .

Susan has been essentially pain-free and diarrhea-free since October 1999 after her liver resection surgery. Regularly scheduled tests seem to indicate that any tumors that remain are not growing so she is "stable".

In December 2004, she was diagnosed as type II diabetic so she has had to manage that as well. In addition she has lost feeling in her feet (neuropathy) but seems to be dealing with that also.

I am lucky to have her. She is amazing . . .

Cancer is a serious health condition . . . but cancer is not your life; it is not the essence of who you are. Do not let cancer define who you are!

Bill

From earliest memory I've always had some degree of gastro-intestinal discomfort and related issues. Because of that, I suppose, it was easy to overlook the gradual increase of problems seemingly related to digestion that became evident in my early 30's. I would struggle along, enduring the bad days, always sure, though, to have a bottle of Pepto—Bismol* in the glove box . . . just in case. This was an incredibly busy time, by anyone's standards, for me and my household. I just didn't have the time to worry about bouts of cramping and diarrhea.

As I moved into my mid-30's, the hurdles of the bad days became more difficult to leap. The pain of cramping overshadowed everything, and I became adept at knowing the locations of all available restrooms whenever I had to be away from home. I would still have stretches of good days, but week after week of profound gastric discomfort was more the norm. Occasionally, the cramping would leave me bed-ridden, and at least once I had family take me to the local hospital emergency room when the pain seemed more than I could bear.

Toward the end of 1993, in my 39th year, debilitating pain and diarrhea became a full time occurrence. I began to see a Gastroenterologist on a regular basis for diagnosis and treatment. My memory of this period is a jumble of tests, pain, dramatic weight loss and endless visits to the bathroom. Mostly I remember long hours huddled in a chair before a front window, watching the rest of the world get on with life. I was completely unable to work by November of that year. Thankfully, I had managed to save a good deal of sick leave. There would be little of that left by the time I was finally able to return to work. Family and friends helped with obligations as I struggled to get a handle on my illness and climb back to good health.

The gastroenterologist I was seeing felt strongly that I had Crohn's Disease, and started me on a regimen of Prednisone. The pain, cramping and diarrhea continued unabated, and it wasn't long before I could not process food at all, having to take in whatever nutrients I could via a liquid diet. Even that did not always stay with me long enough to digest. I fell from a weight of about 180 pounds to 130 pounds. Some friends urged me to be tested for AIDS, I looked that emaciated.

When it became evident to me that the course of prednisone was not having any effect, and when the GI doctor essentially threw up his hands in bewilderment, I contacted a surgeon recommended to me by people I'd come to know in a Crohn's support community. The surgeon scheduled surgery quickly, and in March of 1994 he discovered an orange-sized tumor blocking my digestive tract at the ileocecal valve. It was removed in a right hemi-colectomy procedure, and shown to be carcinoid through pathology testing. The surgeon also found tumor material in the mesentery and liver. Only the material in the mesentery was removed. I felt immensely better within a day of the surgery.

The surgeon recommended I see an oncologist, who I began to see while still recovering at the hospital. The initial course of treatment was a "wait and see" approach. I continued to improve and gain weight. I resumed exercise, and seemed to have regained good health. Throughout the first year or so after surgery the oncologist monitored my blood-serotonin levels, and had me get CAT scans periodically to monitor two small tumors in the liver.

In 1996 my oncologist had me consult with a liver surgeon to discuss the possibility of a liver resection to remove the tumorous area. I went in for surgery late in 1996, but the surgeon did not perform the resection. He told me that he found too many small lesions over practically the whole surface of my liver. He described it as if someone had scattered a handful of rice over the surface of my liver. My oncologist felt that, since surgery was no longer an option,

I should begin chemotherapy treatments. He prescribed a regimen of 5-Flurouracil and Leucovorin once each week. I don't know the dosages. I remained on that protocol for about 3 years, sometime in 1997 until mid-2000, when I requested to be taken off.

At some point after the attempted resection I experienced what my oncologist felt was a "carcinoid crisis". On one particular day I was experiencing particularly severe cramps and light-headedness, and went to the oncology office for a consult with a nurse-practitioner. While in the waiting room I momentarily lost consciousness. My blood pressure was found to be dangerously low (I cannot recall the reading), and so I was given oxygen and an ambulance was called to take me to the hospital. I was kept there for at least several days under observation. My oncologist visited me there and recommended I begin sub-cutaneous Sandostatin® injections.

I then began a daily regimen of the self-injections (I do not remember the dosage) several times each day, until the once-per-month Sandostatin LAR treatment was approved for the public. I started the LAR shots every 28 days at that point. I believe my initial dose was 20mg. At some point between then and now, likely due to my complaints of periodic gastrointestinal discomfort and occasional diarrhea, the dosage was increased to 30mg, where it has remained until present.

In the first years after 2000 my symptoms of carcinoid syndrome (periodic cramping, diarrhea, and occasionally severe fatigue) were beginning to significantly impact my ability to carry out my career as a USPS Letter Carrier. I applied for, and was granted, a disability retirement in 2004.

I have recently moved and am now being cared for at a different oncology office. In the past couple of years I have had increasing bouts of moderate cramping. I have taken the digestive supplement Creon from time-to-time, and am on it now. At my last visit with my oncologist, he told me that he would likely change the frequency of the LAR shots from every 28 days to every 21 days. I am expecting that change with my next scheduled shot in January, 2013.

I really think my coping system is fairly simple and straight-forward. I don't remember ever taking the diagnosis of carcinoid cancer all that seriously, and definitely NOT as a major life-changing event. I recall considering that it was probably going to complicate life somewhat, but I felt so much better immediately after the surgery that removed the bowel-blocking tumor that all I wanted to do was get back to active involvement in life.

As soon as I was cleared and released from the hospital in 1994, I resumed my avid interest in bicycling (albeit more gently at first). Within the year I started exercising again.

The attempted liver resection had a more deleterious effect on me. My spirits flagged, and I recognized that I was in danger of losing my positive edge. I remembered reading about Norman Cousins aiding his healing from a life-threatening illness through watching Marx Brothers movies (humor). I contacted some of my friends and asked them to lend me their favorite funny movies. I feel confident that this and listening to uplifting music brought me around, and I regained my positive approach to managing my illness. This was around 1996.

In the years since I rarely reveal my diagnosis, only because I don't want to be defined by it. My wife and I are gym members, and I work out through resistance and cardio training at least 3 times each week. Without meaning to sound immodest, I definitely feel I'm in better shape than most "healthy" men my age, let alone those battling a cancer diagnosis. I've continued to work at various jobs since retirement, and even ran my own dog walking business for 6 years with my wife. Shortly after moving here to the beach in North Carolina, I took a summer job at a local bicycle shop. Just a few days ago I ordered an inexpensive flute on Amazon.com, and I'm in touch with a teacher . . . just to illustrate my continuing exercises in living and learning. I am not so much engaged in struggling to stay alive as I am just trying to LIVE, and to be MINDFUL of every experience.

This is not to say that I never have moments of fear and disquiet about the possibilities of a long-term illness like carcinoid cancer. I've just been successful, so far, in pushing myself past those momentary fears, and focus on every great thing that's going on in my life (and there are A LOT of great things going on!).

Fear is a darkroom where negatives develop.
—Usman B. Asif

Lawrence W. Chinnery, Sr. (Larry)

My initial symptoms were unexplained falls, weakening of the muscles on the right side of my body; extreme fatigue, muscular aches and pains, abdominal cramping, flu-like muscle aches, occasional serious watery diarrhea, and occasional loss of consciousness, all which began in 1972 or 1976 at the age of 34 or 37 years.

Diagnosis: April 27, 1992 at age 53—Metastatic carcinoid tumors in the liver and spleen (over two dozen), primary not located, and carcinoid syndrome.

Method of diagnoses: Medical work-up, colonoscopy, CT-scan, biopsy and a 5-HIAA by a gastroenterologist

Previous (possible) misdiagnoses:
1972: Undiagnosed
1976: Borderline hypoglycemia
1985: Reactive Airways Dysfunction Syndrome
1988: Post-Polio Syndrome and possible Narcolepsy

I was also told by several physicians over a fifteen-year period (prior to 1992) to see a psychiatrist—that it was "all in my head"—even when I coughed up blood in their office.

Treatments: I completed thirty-six courses of chemotherapy (one course consists of intravenous infusion for four or five contiguous days) between June 1992 and the spring of 1997. I have also self-injected somatostatin analogue since June 1992, later switching to Sandostatin LAR®. The above two therapies completely eliminated all visible tumors from various scans by the spring of 1997.

By 1999, various scans began to again show several large tumors in the right lobe of my liver. In the summer of 2001, the pains began to become significant again. In anticipation of performing a radio-frequency ablation, surgeons (at the National Institutes of Health) performed exploratory laparoscopic surgery on me, but determined the number of tumors in my liver to be too numerous to continue with the RFA. Chemoembolization was advised instead.

I completed a chemoembolization on May 1, 2002. It took me about six weeks to recover from that procedure—and feeling better than I had in years—just in time for . . . a Phase II trial of Gleevec® for carcinoid in 2002. I had to discontinue this therapy and trial in early 2003 as I experienced two severe infections—a skin infection but then also Clostridium difficile in my intestine. What fun to have to take an ambulance to the hospital just after two feet of snow had fallen!

In the fall of 2002 I learned that the carcinoid had entered into my bones. I began to be in severe pain from the bone metastases in spring 2003, and this pain continued to develop into the summer, at which time I was using very significant quantities of opiates just to "get through" the days and nights. In November of 2002, I was started on infusions of Zometa® for bone strengthening.

In June 2003, it was determined that the extent of my bone metastases included my femurs, hips, entire spine, shoulders and ribs. I, apparently, might have also fractured my left femur; all of which accounted for the severe pain. I, therefore, underwent external beam radiation of my left hip.

Soon thereafter, I underwent infusions of Samarium-153 to abate the pain of the bone metastases. This has proven to be a very effective treatment for me as most of the pain abated within 24 hours. Two months later (September 2003) I determined that the use of one or two Vioxx® took any "residual" pain away. In February 2004 the pain had once again gained a hold of me, and so I had a second Samarium-153 infusion.

Because of continued metastatic tumor growth (liver, spleen, and bones), I began searching for a systemic treatment in late 2003. In April 2004 I began taking injections of interferon (Intron A®) in addition to the Zometa® and Sandostatin LAR®. By May I had to stop the interferon injections due to unexplained bleeding and fatigue. I restarted the Interferon a few weeks later and continued this therapy into July, 2004.

Onset of Diabetes: In mid-May 2004, and probably due to the years of Sandostatin® treatment, I began treatment with insulin and other meds for type II diabetes.

Another Chemotherapy regime: In August 2004 I began a new chemotherapy regime on a twenty-eight day cycle—14 days on and 14 days off. During days 1-14, I took Xeloda® (pills). During days 10-14, I took Kytril® and Temodar® as well. But because my blood counts (particularly the platelets) became so low in late September 2004, I had to put additional chemotherapy and diabetes treatments on hold so I could have a platelet blood transfusion

Subdural Hematoma: After several more blood transfusions, I was hospitalized for several days in early November 2004 because a brain CT-scan showed that I had developed a subdural hematoma in my right front brain. Initially this was thought to be very serious; but it was determined, via other CT-scans that this "problem" would probably right itself without surgery. I began monitoring this condition with MRIs of my brain every six weeks. After several months they continued to shrink.

Skull Tumor: Unfortunately, the MRI also showed new metastatic disease in the left posterior skull. This was confirmed by an OctreoScan® done in February 2005. I am left with the question: What to do with this latest invasion of my space? My Chromogranin A, over time, had dropped, probably meaning that my tumor load has decreased significantly. Unfortunately by February 2005, an OctreoScan® indicated massive uptake in both liver nodes, left shoulder and my skull.

Additional tumor Load: In early May 2005, I began having extreme chest pains. An abdominal and chest CT-scan indicated an increase in the tumor in the left lobe of my liver. I was scheduled for a second chemoembolization in mid-July. However, because the mid-chest pain stopped the second week of July, I cancelled the chemoembolization and undertook more systemic chemotherapy using Xeloda®. Because I fell asleep for most of each day (for several weeks) after one round of Xeloda®, it was stopped.

September 2005: The pains in my lower spine and hips have returned with a vengeance. I was able to take another Samarium[153]

infusion soon but it provided only a couple weeks of relief instead of the 6 and 9 months the earlier treatments provided.

I then got a little more pain relief from laparoscopic surgery to remove my gall bladder. At that time my veins had become so hard to find that I finally gave in and had a port installed in my upper chest. Eventually I admitted to my wife that I should have done this 15 years earlier as it sure made blood tests and intravenous chemotherapy easier.

Winter 2005-2006: Fitting my motto of "we can still have some more fun yet", my wife and I took a western Caribbean cruise. I rented an electric scooter that was delivered to the dock.

My oncologist proposed that we try some newer biochemical therapies approved for some other cancers but not yet for carcinoid. The Avastin* turned me into a kind of zombie. I perked up soon after stopping it. Then we went to straight Xeloda* without adding Temodar* this time. I was feeling a lot better and we even planned two vacation trips for June.

But then, oops, my blood counts were too low so I had to take a break from chemotherapy. I would check back every week or so but still—no go.

Then came June 1, 2006. That day the doc ordered additional blood tests and informed my wife and me that my bone marrow was now "shot", presumably due to the bone metastases.

He advised hospice. After about 10 days of home hospice visits, I was taken (by a bumpy and jerky ambulance!) to inpatient hospice.

Linda speaking now: Larry chose inpatient hospice so (1) I would not have the memory of him dying at home and (2) he could have better pain control. He entered a coma on June 20 and died on June 21.

Lawrence's journey was excerpted with permission of his wife, Linda Silversmith, from his personal blog. Linda added the update from September 2005 to June 2006.

http://noids.netfirms.com/html/personal_.html

Larry was active in the carcinoid community, putting on many regional carcinoid presentations and educating others. Another of his favorite mottoes was "keep on keeping on". The last update to his website was in September 2005. Larry Chinnery Sr., sadly passed away on June 21, 2006.

❖

"Inaction breeds doubt and fear. Action breeds confidence and courage. If you want to conquer fear, do not sit home and think about it. Go out and get busy."

—Dale Carnegie

Self Help for Managing Diarrhea

Causes of Diarrhea:

Diarrhea is one of the most troublesome symptoms persons with NETs have to deal with. It can be caused by surgery (short-gut syndrome), where a part of the intestine is removed due to disease involvement and the two ends sutured back together. This removal and re-joining (anastomosis) of the intestine can lead to a rapid transit time of food that is ready to be absorbed by the body. The shortened bowel can lead to diarrhea. (There are many other causes of diarrhea in NETs but are beyond the scope of this book. Your doctor can help evaluate the cause and recommend treatment). It is not uncommon for some people to have up to 20 or more bowel movements in a day, especially if not on Sandostatin˚ or other medications to control diarrhea. This obviously can lead to dehydration and all that accompanies this condition: fatigue, weight loss, muscle wasting, inability to absorb nutrients, dizziness and even syncope (fainting). If diarrhea is not treated, it can lead to death.

High fiber or greasy, spicy, sweet foods or raw fruits and vegetables may be the cause.

Many are lactose intolerant in addition to the food sensitivities.

When Diarrhea is a Problem

Maintain good hydration. Ten to twelve ounces per day, minimum.

This includes diluted fruit juices, weak tea, flat lemon lime soda, diluted sports drinks, clear soups and broths, Horchata (a Mexican drink found in most grocery stores) made with rice milk and containing nutmeg which is good for diarrhea.

Eat small frequent meals.

Eat slowly and chew your food well, at least 20-30 chews so your food is almost liquid. This will help start the digestive process and your gastrointestinal tract will not have to work as hard to assimilate nutrients.

Avoid foods that can make diarrhea worse:
- Caffeinated foods and drinks (chocolate, coffee, tea, some sodas.
- Spicy foods such as chili, garlic or other highly seasoned foods.
- Concentrated sweets (cookies, cake, candy) et al.
- Greasy or fatty foods (fried foods, full fat cheese, ice cream, potato or corn chips, et al.
- Fluid milk (yogurt is usually okay.
- Foods high in insoluble fiber such as bran cereal, fruit skins, raw vegetables, nuts, seeds, popcorn, and gas formers such as beans, cabbage, broccoli, cauliflower)

What to Eat
BRATT diet: bananas, rice, applesauce, toast, tea.

This diet is low in protein and should not be consumed for more than a day or two. You may add boiled chicken to this diet for added protein or Tofu if you are Vegetarian.

Other foods you can eat: flavored gelatin, yogurt with live cultures or take a Probiotic capsule. There are many on the market and some can be expensive but are worth it to establish normal flora in the intestine which will help with diarrhea.

White fish is a good choice, hard boiled eggs unless you are Vegan, cream of wheat or rice, rice cakes, sweet potatoes, broth, plain crackers, cooked carrots, potatoes without the skin.

Gradually advance food intake until your diarrhea is under control. If you cannot control it and become symptomatic, go to your nearest emergency room or call 911!

Laughter is always the best medicine . . . unless you have diarrhea.

—unknown

Notes:

Tips for Maintaining Weight

A lot of us eat small meals versus large and have problems with diarrhea due to short-gut syndrome from our surgeries. It is very important to keep weight on and a challenge for many.

What we choose to eat matters more than usual when the amount we eat is small. Improved nutrition will help you feel better as will drinking plenty of water to combat fatigue. The majority of persons with fatigue are dehydrated, especially with diarrhea and/or lack of an appetite due to illness or opiates. Be sure to have your thyroid function assessed if you have fatigue that is not related to dehydration.

Start with protein foods. Fruits and vegetables contain a lot of valuable nutrients, but they can be light on calories. They also contain fiber and for those with a history of bowel obstructions, it is extremely important to maintain a low fiber diet. Foods high in fats and sugar will add extra calories, but not as many nutrients.

Find a Balance

Adding a little extra butter or olive oil to meals adds calories without adding bulk. Liquid calories can also be easy to add between meals. They don't make you feel full, yet can add extra calories.

Guidelines

Plan a daily or even a week's menu in advance.

Make every bite count; choose foods high in calories and protein and low in fiber.

Pack snacks to keep on hand at all times.

Eat at least 1/3 of calorie and protein needs at breakfast.

Eat 5-6 small meals per day as tolerated.

Don't be afraid to try something new, as this might help your appetite.

Exercise as tolerated but do not if you have symptoms such as fatigue, dizziness, or any problems that will be aggravated by exercise. You can exercise in a chair (upper body movements such as weight lifting or paper plate exercise).

YOU ARE YOUR BEST ADVOCATE AND KNOW WHAT DOES AND DOES NOT WORK!

Ideas to Add Calories

Peanut butter, unless allergic (with or without jelly).

Nuts: as a snack or as a butter (walnut or almond, hemp.

Sprinkle hemp, chia, or sesame seeds on soups, salads, eggs, or whatever you see fit and that works for you.

Add protein powders or dry milk to foods to boost protein content.

Liquid calories as in smoothies.

Juice, may be diluted or add to smoothies or other liquid supplements.

Milk unless lactose intolerant. Use alternatives to milk if allergic or intolerant to milk, such as soy, almond milk, coconut milk.

Kefir or low fat buttermilk.

Milkshakes or malts with added ingredients.to boost caloric value.

Ensure, Boost, Peptamin, Carnation instant breakfast or what appeals to you.

Try adding a little of these to your foods to boost calories:

- Cheese
- Butter
- Extra virgin olive oil
- MCT oil
- Flaxseed oil
- Udo's Oil (may cause diarrhea if taken on an empty stomach

These are suggestions. Check with your doctor or other medical provider before implementing any of the above recommendations!

Carcinoid Crisis:
Prevention and Treatment

The gravest, life-threatening event facing NETs patients is carcinoid crisis. It can occur with physical exams, especially if the examiner is palpating deeply over the liver lobes, during dental procedures, anesthesia induction, surgical procedures and even due to strongly emotional events.

It does not matter what type of tumor a NETs patient has, they are all subject to carcinoid crisis. To date, a standardized dose of octreotide to prevent crisis has not been firmly established, but there are guidelines that have been developed based on the experience of hundreds of surgeries from centers all over the world.

Copying and showing this information to your physicians before any medical procedure could save your life.

A Definition:
- Immediate onset of a debilitating and life-threatening condition associated with carcinoid syndrome
- May occur spontaneously or may be precipitated by anesthesia, chemotherapy, infection, stress, catecholamines, tumor manipulation or embolization procedures
- Symptoms include prolonged severe flushing, diarrhea, hypotension, tachycardia, severe dyspnea, peripheral cyanosis and sometimes hemodynamic instability
- Appropriate precautions include immediate octreotide therapy and close monitoring before, during and after surgical treatment.
-

—Oberg K. Williams Textbook of Endocrinology;
10th Ed. Saunders; 2003 pp.1857-1876

The following is an email transcript (edited for punctuation) from Dr. Eugene Woltering MD of the Ochsner Medical Center in Kenner, Louisiana:

Date: Wed, 6 Jan 2010 16:57:19—0600
OUR APPROACH TO THE PREVENTION AND TREATMENT OF INTRAOPERATIVE CARCINOID CRISIS

The NOLANETs group uses this—others use less; we can't speak to their results—but even with these "higher than others" type dosing we have had 2 carcinoid crises out of about 300 major cytoreductive surgical procedures.

Two hours before surgery we give 500 micrograms of octreotide acetate aqueous IV push. To prevent nausea we often pretreat folks with an antiemetic before the octreotide IV push.

Then we start a 500 microgram per hour IV infusion of octreotide acetate. Start this immediately after the IV push and continue infusion during and after surgery

Depending on the severity and duration of surgery, taper the infusion over 1-4 hours. For colonoscopy, taper over approximately 1 hour. After huge liver cases taper over 12-24 hours. **If the patient crashes, don't use pressors**: they can cause degranulation of the amine producing cells. Only use pressors as the last resort if the following regimen fails: Use IV fluids and 1-5 mg. bolus of octreotide (can repeat every 10 minutes if needed). For cases of malignant hyperthermia (very rare) we use dantrolene in normal doses

I hope this helps. If all else fails print this out sheet and hand it to your anesthesia person along with my cell phone number: 504-884-3555

If your physicians get into trouble have them call me on my cell phone day or night.

Eugene A. Woltering MD FACS

The James D. Rives Professor of Surgery and Neurosciences
LSUHSC Department of Surgery
New Orleans, LA 70112
504-884-3555-cell

Definition of a Pressor

A vasopressor (or just "pressor") raises blood pressure by constricting blood vessels. Drugs such as dopamine and norepinephrine are used in the emergency or operating room as well as ICU if a patient starts to become hypotensive, usually from sepsis (blood infection) or organ failure as a result of it, or severe trauma.

Malignant hyperthermia may be part of carcinoid crisis and this will need to be addressed as well by the professionals caring for you. (ISI, 2013).

Published Prophylactic Treatment:

Prophylactic administration of octreotide must be given by continuous intravenous infusion at a dose of 50 µg/h for 12 hours prior to and at least 48 hours after the procedure to prevent a cardiovascular carcinoid crisis.

Ramage JK et al. Guidelines for the management of gastroenteropancreatic neuroendocrine (including carcinoid) tumours. Gut. 2005;54(suppl 4);iv1-16

Lots of folks confuse bad management with destiny.
—Kin Hubbard

References

AARP, Magazine, Quality of Life., 2007; 30-32

Adler, M., MD, 2013, personal communication

Alschuler, ND, Lise; Gazella, Karolyn A. "Five to Thrive: Your Cutting Edge Cancer Prevention Plan" 2011 El Segundo, CA Active Interest Media Inc.

Anthony, L.B., MD, editor, Carcinoid Tumors and Carcinoid Syndrome, 2004, 3-11

Anthony L. MD, and Vinik A.I., MD, 2011,Consensus Guidelines for the Diagnosis and Management of Neuroendocrine Tumors 2010; 713-715.

Anderson JL, Dodman S, Kopelman M, Fleming A. Patient information recall in a rheumatology clinic. Rheumatol Rehabil 1979;18: 245-55

Barden, Catherine B., Fahey III, Thomas J., Kvols, Larry K. (2002) Neuroendocrine Tumors of the Gastrointestinal Tract, Gastrointestinal Oncology; Principles and Practice Lippincott, Williams, and Wilkins

Bates, Barbara, M.D. (1979). A Guide to Physical Examination. Second Edition, Philadelphia, Toronto: J. B. Lippincott Company. Chapter 12; The Abdomen

Brandon, Barbara "Survive Your Cancer" Survivor's Wisdom 2003

Carcinoid Cancer Awareness Network www.carcinoidawareness.org Bob & Maryann Wahmann, Founders and Editors

Carcinoid Cancer Foundation www.carcinoid.org Grace Goldstein, COO & Editor

Caring for Carcinoid www.caringforcarcinoid.org Nancy Lindholm, Founder & Director

Chobanian, Sarkis J. MD and Van Ness, Michael M. MD. (1988). Manual Of Clinical Problems In Gastroenterology. Carcinoid Tumors and The Carcinoid Syndrome. Lippincott Williams & Wilkins. pp. 105-108

Cohen, Elizabeth, CNN Medical Correspondent. (2010). The Empowered Patient. New York: Ballantine Books. pp. 57-58

Cure Magazine www.curetoday.com Dallas TX Cure Media Group

Dachs, Robert, MD (December, 2001) "Eleven Common Myths About Pain Control" Emergency Medicine Vol. 33, No. 12, p. 19

Dewey, Michael. (February 28, 2013) Bone Health News by AlageCal, Issue 173.

Dollinger, M., M.D., Rosenbaum, EH, M.D., Cable, G. (1997) Everyone's Guide to Cancer Therapy, Revised 3rd edition, Somerville House Book, Andrews McMeel Publishing, Kansas City pp. 125-160; 391-396

Engstrom, Paul "Russell Portenoy: Giving Patients Relief" Cure Magazine Special Issue, Cure Media Group, October 2008

Emeka, Mauris L. Cancer's Best Medicine, A self-help and wellness guide 2008, 9-25

Epstein, Lew, et al. Trusting You Are Loved—Practices for Partnership. Partnership Foundation, 1999

Fauci, Braunwald, Isselbacher, Wilson Martin, Kasper, Hauser, Longo. (2000). Harrison's Principles of Internal Medicine 14th Edition Companion Handbook. McGraw—Hill Companies, ISBN 0-07-021530-8, Carcinoid syndrome, diarrhea from, pp. 82, 87, Carcinoid tumor, pp. 320, treatment of, pp. 320, 321, 343

Fisher, G. MD, Kulke, Clinical Trials, Conference, 2013, San Francisco Conference, Helen Diller, UCSF, NET Patient Kickoff Conference

Fortson, Leigh "Embrace, Release, Heal" 2011 Boulder, Co Sounds True, Inc.

Francis, M.Sc., Raymond "Never Fear Cancer Again—How to Prevent and Reverse Cancer" 2011, Deersfield Beach, FL Health Communications Inc.

Goldfinger, SE, MD, Strosberg, Jonathan R, MD.(October 31, 2012). Clinical Features of the Carcinoid Syndrome. http://www.uptodate.com/contents/clinical-features-of-the-carcinoid-syndrome

Gray, H. F.R.S., Ed. By Lewis, W.H., B.S., M.D., Mason, Karl E. (July, 1944). Gray's Anatomy of The Human Body. Lea and Febiger, Philadelphia, 24th ed. pp. 1121-1223

Grotto, David, (2011). 101 Foods That Could Save Your Life. New York: Bantam Mass Market Edition. pp. 7, 64; 352-354

Kulke, MH. (2003). Neuroendocrine Tumors: Clinical Presentation and Management of Localized Disease. Cancer Treatment Reviews, 29:5 pp. 363-70

Kvols, LK. (1994). Metastatic Carcinoid Tumors and the Malignant Carcinoid Syndrome. Annals of the New York Academy of Science, pp. 733: 464

Lie, JP. (1982). Carcinoid tumor, Carcinoid Syndrome, and Carcinoid Heart Disease. Prim Cardiol 8: p.163

Longo, Dan; et al., editors "Harrison's Gastroenterology & Hepatology" 2010 McGraw-Hill Publications pp. 533-551

Longo, Dan; et al., editors "Harrison's Principles of Internal Medicine" 18th Edition 2012 McGraw-Hill Publications

Maraire, Greta, RD, MA, Nutrition lecture, UCSF. 2013, Live Conference, NET Patient Kickoff ConferenceMamikunian, Gregg et. al; InterScience Institute GI Council "Neuroendocrine Tumors: A Comprehensive Guide to Diagnosis and Management" InterScience Institute, 2009

Mamikunian, Paris; Ardill, Joy E.; O'Dorisio, Thomas M.; Krutzik, Siegfried R.; Vinik, Aaron I.; Go, Vay Liang W.; Armstrong, Lee; Mamikunian, Gregg; Woltering, Eugene A.(October, 2011) Validation of Neurokinin A Assays in the United States and Europe. Pancreas 40, Number 7, pp. 1000-1004

McGuire LC. Remembering what the doctor said: organization and older adults' memory for medical information. Exp Aging Res 1996;22: 403-28

Mechanick, Jeffrey I, MD "Nutrition and Diet for Carcinoid Patients: An Interview with Mechanick, MD Jeffrey I. Carcinoid Cancer Foundation (Retrieved February 2010) www.carcinoid.org/content/nutrition-and-diet-carcinoid-patients-interview-jeffrey-i-mechanick-md

Miller, Michael Craig, M.D., (2011) Harvard Mental Health Letter, Harvard Medical School http://www.health.harvard.edu/special_health_reports/Understanding_Depression

Modlin, IM, Kidd, M, Latich, I, et al. (2006) Current Status of Gastrointestinal Carcinoids. Clinical Gastroenterology and Hepatology. 4: pp. 526-547

Modlin I M, Lye, K D, Kidd M. A 5-decade analysis of 13,715 carcinoid tumors. Cancer. 2003; 97:934-959

Mukherjee MD, Siddhartha "The Emperor of All Maladies" 2010 New York, NY Simon & Schuster

National Cancer Institute. What You Need to Know About Cancer. September, Retrieved September 2001, www.cancer.gov/cancertopics/wyntk/overview/allpages

National Cancer Institute. (April 2011) Eating Hints: Before, During, and After Cancer Treatment. NIH No. 11-2079. pp. 20, 21, 27, 37, 39, 41

National Cancer Institute. General Information About Gastrointestinal Carcinoid Tumors. Retrieved June 2012, www.cancer.gov/cancertopics/pdq/treatment/gastrointestinalcarcinoid/Patient

National Institutes of Health. Inside the Cell. Retrieved July 18, 2012, from www.publications.nigms.nih.gov/insidethecell

Net Cancer Day www.netcancerday.org/learn-more/what-is-net-cancer 2011 World NET Community

Netter, F.K. M.D. (1990). Atlas of Human Anatomy. Ciba-Geigy Corp. Summit, NJ, 3rd Ed. pp. 220-314

Nuland MD, Sherwin B. "How We Die Reflections of Life's Final Chapter" 1995 New York, NY Vintage Books

Nutrition Action Healthletter, Center for Science in the Public Interest, Washington, D.C. 2012

Oberg, K.E. Department of Endocrine Oncology, University Hospital, Uppala, Sweden. (2012, May). The Management of Neuroendocrine Tumors: Current and Future Medical Therapy Options. Clinical Oncology, 24:4, pages 282-293

Perez, E.A., Koniaris, L.G., Snell, S.E., Gutierrez, J.C., Sumner, W.E.3rd., Lee, D.J., Hodgson, N.C., Livingstone, A.S., & Franceschi, D. 7201 carcinoids: increasing incidence overall and disproportionate mortality in the elderly. World Journal of Surgery, 2007, 31(5): 1022-1030

Peeke, Pamela MD, July-August, AARP Magazine, 2007

Pommier, Rodney MD. (2010, October). Management of Hepatic Metastasis—Making The Right Choice. Neuroendocrine Tumor Symposium Syllabus

Pommier, Rodney, MD. (2012, March 20). Carcinoid Crisis and Surgery. Retrieved October 11, 2012, from: www.carcinoid. org/sites/default/files/Carcioid%20NET%20Cancer%20 Specialist%20Rodney%20F.%20Pommier%20on%20 Carcinoid%20Crisis%20and%20Surger.pdf

Pommier, Rodney, MD, FACS "The Role of Surgery and Chemoembolization in the Management of Carcinoid" presented at California Carcinoid Fighters Conference, October 25, 2003, http://www.carcinoid.org/content/role-surgery-and-chemoembolization-management-carcinoid

Qian Y, Fan JG. Obesity, fatty liver and liver cancer. Hepatobiliary Pancreat Dis Int. 2005 May;4(2):173-7.

Servan-Schreiber, David "Anticancer—A New Way" 2009 New York, NY Penguin Books Ltd.

Shelton BK. Intestinal obstruction. AACN Clin Issues. 1999;10(4):478-491

Steele, Teresa J, MSN, RD. (August 2010). Vitamin B12 Deficiency Clinician Reviews. Vol 20, No. 8 pp.16-19

Stronge, RL et al. "A rapid rise in circulating pancreastatin in response to somatostatin analogue therapy is associated with poor survival in patients with neuroendocrine tumours" Annals of Clinical Biochemistry November 2008 45:560-566

Thernstrom, M. (2010) The Pain Chronicles. New York: Farrar, Straus and Giroux, pp. 282-299

United States and Europe Pancreas Journal Volume 40, Number 7, October 2011, pp 1000-1004

Van Ness MD, Michael M., (Author), Chobanian MD, Sarkis J (Editor) "Manual of Clinical Problems in Gastroenterology" 1994 Boston, MA Little Brown & Company

Vinik, Aaron I., MD, PhD et al. "NANETs Consensus Guidelines for the Diagnosis of Neuroendocrine Tumor"

Vinik AI and Gonzales MR, Endocrnol Metab Clin No. Am, 2011; 44.1:10-63

Vinik, Aaron I., Woltering, Eugene A., O'Dorisio, Thomas M. Go, Vay Liang W., Mamijunian, Gregg (2012) "Neuroendocrine Tumors, A Comprehensive Guide to Diagnosis and Management. Inter Science Institute

Warner, Richard R.P., MD, retrieved December, 2012, from: http://www.carcinoidinfo.info/monitor.htm   www.nanets.net/pdfs/pancreas/03.pdf www.cancer.gov NIH/NCI "General Information About Gastrointestinal Carcinoid Tumors" modified June 2012 www.vitamindcouncil.org/about-vitamin-d/how-to-get-your-vitamin-d/vitamin-d-supplementation/

Index

V

Vitamin D3 46
Vomiting 35

W

Weight Loss 35
Weight Maintenance 211
Wellness Community 85